LOSING TIM

The Life and Death of an American Contractor in Iraq

A Memoir

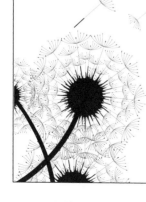

JANET BURROWAY

FOREWORD BY JONATHAN SHAY

Think Piece Publishing | *Singular Voices. Social Issues.*
MINNEAPOLIS

Grateful acknowledgment is made to the following for permission to reprint previously published material: Excerpt from "A Variation on 'To Say to Go To Sleep'" from THE COMPLETE POEMS by Randall Jarrell. Copyright © 1969, renewed 1997 by Mary von S. Jarrell. Reprinted by permission of Farrar, Straus and Giroux, LLC. BEHIND BLUE EYES. Words and Music by PETER TOWNSHEND © 1971 (Renewed) FABU-LOUS MUSIC LTD. Published by FABULOUS MUSIC LTD. Administered in the USA and Canada by SPIRIT ONE MUSIC (BMI) o/b/o SPIRIT SERVICES HOLDINGS, S.à.r.l., SUOLUBAF MUSIC and ABKCO MUSIC INC., 85 Fifth Avenue, New York, NY 10003 International Copyright Secured All Rights Reserved Used By Permission.

Gratitude to the following people who granted us permission to quote from their personal correspondence: Tobyn Alexander Eysselinck, Major Robert Jones, Birgitt Eysselinck, and Gary Pitts.

ISBN: 978-0-9892352-3-5

Printed in the United States of America
Designed by Mayfly Design and Typeset in Adobe Garamond Pro
First Printing: 2014

18 17 16 15 14   5 4 3 2 1

Think Piece Publishing
Singular Voices. Social Issues.
www.thinkpiecepublishing.com

JUL − − 2014

For Tim

Captain, Ranger, Paratrooper, husband, father, brother, hunter,
contractor for humanitarian mine removal in Iraq,
Republican, romantic, idealist, perfectionist,
gun nut, my firstborn,
my baby.

FOREWORD

by Jonathan Shay

There is a lot of pain in this book, but the beauty and artistry of the writing make it endurable without sentimental slight of hand. To me, the pain recalls Homer's *Iliad,* in which, as James Tatum provocatively puts it in *The Mourner's Song,* "the beauty [of the poetry] is in the killing,"

Losing Tim's author is the mother of Timothy Eysselinck, an accomplished US Army Captain with both Ranger and Airborne training, who leaves the Army to work as a contractor so he can continue the humanitarian demining he has been doing as an officer—the Army had shed demining to a private corporation. After a period in Iraq, he quits in disgust and rage at his employer's financial corruption and wantonness toward human life. Tim returns home to his wife and small children, where a scant two month later he kills himself with one of his own guns. It is not only Janet Burroway who has lost Tim, but also his wife, his children, his friends—as has the Army, which wanted him back, and the nation, which can ill afford to lose people of high talent and high principles *together.*

Reading this book, it is inevitable that those readers, who knew or knew of the late Army Colonel Ted Westhusing, would flash on him. Tim and Ted were cut from the same cloth, passionately aspiring fully to live American soldierly ideals, and both, in my view, were deeply soul-wounded when they discovered that those with authority over them did not. Both had a giant-sized sense of responsibility and felt tainted by the corruption and callous careerism they saw around them and above them—and both fell into despair. I recall that almost instantly after Westhusing's death there was disparaging chatter on military sites that he was "too tightly wound," as if living up to Army principles is a form of mental defect.

In case you are wondering if there was a contagion or copycat element to Tim's suicide, it happened more than a year *before* Westhusing's.

Moral injury occurs when there is a betrayal of what's right in a high stakes situation by someone in legitimate authority. Shortly before his suicide, Tim told his wife he was "tired of being the bad man," manifestly his own judgment of himself, since no one who knew or worked with him (or for him) shared it. Despair kills. The person in despair loses hope of *ever* inhabiting virtue. Despair and suicidality are consequences of moral injury, as, surprisingly, so is shame. "I'm ashamed to be an American"—Tim's words, not long before his suicide, from this deeply patriotic Army officer.

So there you have my conjecture on the "why?" question that those left behind ask about every suicide. No one has asked "why?" more persistently and more poignantly than the author, Tim's mother and biographer. She takes us with her with warmth and intelligence, steadily, but gently and quite unobtrusively through fourteen different explicit or implicit theories by my count of why people take their own lives. Only a reader with a professional vested interest, like me, would ever think to count them up.

Finally, a word about contractors returning to America from warzones overseas. Most are prior-service military veterans, some of whom will have suffered psychological and moral injury in their prior service, in addition to whatever wounds they take on as contractors.

Morally injured veterans are vulnerable to suicide and domestic violence, and also to recruitment by tight criminal, or coercive religious or political groups. The historical record is clear: German WWI veterans who were demobilized *together* and returned together to the town in which their division was raised, generally settled peacefully back into civilian society, even when their home towns were now on the other side of newly drawn national borders. However, members of special *Reichsheer* formations, which were manned by volunteers from regular army units and were demobilized *as individuals* and scattered to the winds—these elite veterans were drawn to paramilitary gangs.

Why raise this historical curiosity here? Because we in America have a sociologically analogous situation with repatriated "trigger-puller" contractors, many special operations troops from the current theaters of war, who have neither home station to return to, nor military unit association, nor clear cut VA eligibility for healthcare and disability pension benefits.

Who will offer social support and mental health services to contractor veterans? Obviously, not all psychologically and morally injured military contractors will ask for help. But as a matter of public policy, it will be a *very* good investment to make them eligible to receive it, without a lot of hoops to jump through. The contracting firms are supposedly obligated to provide medical and disability benefits to injured former employees. Whether or not current law can be construed to compel these firms to provide such coverage—or their insurers to honor it—I regard it as *very* imprudent for us as a nation to rely upon such legal ambiguities.

Tim turned the explosive energies unleashed by moral injury upon himself, and we might suppose that his fine and upright character would foreclose his turning it upon others in violent criminal or political ways. But established adult good character is NOT unchanging and immovable as stone. Morally injured, repatriated contractors with military skills of the sort that Tim possessed will be denied health and pension benefits to *our* peril, as much as theirs.

It has been a pleasure and a privilege to get to know the author through this candid and very personal narrative. Her candor about herself with the reader reminds me of the candor between close friends reunited after, say, 50 years separation. (Having just passed my 50th college reunion, that is the parallel that springs to mind.) I had not known Janet Burroway or her work prior to the publisher requesting a blurb for the dust jacket, but having read the manuscript in its entirety, I offered to write this foreword instead.

———

Jonathan Shay is a clinical psychiatrist whose treatment of combat trauma suffered by Vietnam veterans combined with his critical and imaginative interpretations of the ancient accounts of battle described in Homer's *Iliad* and *Odyssey* are deepening our understanding of the effects of warfare on the individual. His book, *Achilles in Vietnam: Combat Trauma and the Undoing of Character* (1994), draws parallels between the depiction of the epic warrior-hero Achilles and the experiences of individual veterans whom he treated at a Boston-area Veterans Affairs' Outpatient Clinic. Reading the poem through the lens of modern experience, Shay rediscovers important nuances that traditional scholarship has often understated in the classical text, particularly that the *Iliad* is fundamentally a story about the frequently contentious relationship between soldiers and their leaders. In *Odysseus in America: Combat Trauma and the Trials of Homecoming* (2002), using Odysseus as metaphor, Shay focuses on the veteran's experience upon returning from war and highlights the role of military policy in promoting the mental and physical safety of soldiers. A passionate advocate for veterans and committed to minimizing future psychological trauma, Shay strives for structural reform of the ways the U.S. armed forces are organized, trained, and counseled.

If you've never wept and want to, have a child.

—DAVID FOSTER WALLACE,
"INCARNATIONS OF BURNED CHILDREN"

What's to be done with the lost, the dead, but write them into being?

—HILARY MANTEL,
GIVING UP THE GHOST

In every story I tell comes a point where I can see no further.

—ANNE CARSON,
"ON HOMO SAPIENS"

1.

Every suicide is a suicide bomber. The intention may be absolutely other—a yearning for peace, the need to escape, even a desire to spare the family. Nevertheless the shrapnel flies.

———

My husband Peter and I had been to a movie. We'd barely stowed our things when the phone rang. Our daughter-in-law Birgitt, halfway round the world in Africa, said, "Didn't you get my messages?" I fumbled, apologizing, "Oh, I hadn't checked." Her voice blank, Birgitt said, "Tim has shot himself," and I replied, "How badly is he hurt?" I saw him hunting on a game reserve near their home in Namibia. My first image was of a bullet hole in his foot. I remember that in this image the foot was, absurdly, wearing a sock. I called to Peter, "Get on the phone! Tim has shot himself!" and he picked up the receiver and said, "How badly is he hurt?"

Yet it was not many seconds before both of us took in the mortal contraction, "He's gone," and not many seconds after that when we understood that this going had been his intention. In some acid reflux of emotion I said to myself: *I knew it; more than once he said he would die young; I won't mind much.*

Later I indicted myself for that grotesque rupture of self-knowledge. Later still I recounted it to a few close friends who had wandered into the topic of denial; it stopped the conversation cold.

———

The end of the story, I told my students, is the most important part. We can't help it. It happens willy-nilly—the last sentence echoes backward through all the rest. You cast back over the scenes to understand how the parts fit together, how character and chance and history converged, what clues you missed, how differently this or that scene looks in the light of what happened after. It isn't a question of drama or surprise, I said, but resonance and rightness. Because we readers *will* look for whatever we mean by "meaning."

Now I see that, working backward from the end of Tim's story, trying to understand it, I run the danger of reading suicide into every incident, distorting the meaning of his life toward its heart-rending close. I accept that part of the job of grieving is to search, re-search, try to reach some minimally satisfying sense of why it must end this way. What is hard is that all the old stories have changed their point as well. Every one of my mother-memories is skewed and spoiled.

A small instance: I sat on a step in the breakfast room in my robe, an abounding ashtray beside me, waiting up for 17-year-old Tim, to whom I had recently given his first car. He appeared at 4 a.m., shoes in hand. I flipped the switch and scared the daylights out of him, might as well have brandished a rolling pin like a shrew in a cartoon. Next day I spoke of it to a friend who put an end to such scenes by saying (always the punch line of this anecdote), "Not many of them kill themselves. And no mother ever prevented it by waiting up."

———

Tim was born in a clinic in Ghent, Belgium, peopled by nuns in winged wimples and run by a revered doctor who never took a day off from delivering babies, whose name I have now forgotten but whose spatulate, leviathan hands I remember for their surprising delicacy. Walter Eysselinck and I had met at the Yale School of Drama, had been married by William Sloane Coffin in the Yale chapel, and two years later had come back to Walter's hometown, where he was directing for Flemish television. I was twenty-seven, a foreigner with only the rudiments of the language, painfully polite with the mother-in-law we had displaced, living in the Bauhaus home where my husband had grown up. I had dutifully gone for checkups at the awesome doctor's clinic and attended classes with the "kinesthetician" who would, in a remarkably forward-looking practice, be present at the birth.

But I did not recognize labor when it happened. I was ten days overdue and made of lead. I woke with a crippling backache. Walter made some demand. I reacted, we quarreled, and he slammed out. By the time I realized I was in labor, called a cab, and got myself and my suitcase down the stairs, he was on the train to Brussels and unreachable. By the time he was located and made it back to Ghent, I was in hard labor. He hovered behind my shoulder. Having been admirably prepared, I was unprepared. Episiotomy and forceps were required. Afterward Walter focused on the wording and the font of the birth announcement, while I swallowed my dismay that we had spoiled the irretrievable event.

By contrast, Tim's little brother Tobyn Alexander (known as Toby until he was eight years old, and Alex after that) was born at home on Guy Fawkes Day in the smallest room of a ramshackle house under the Sussex downs in England, where the district nurse had advised me to "make a hundred balls of cotton wool and bake them in a biscuit tin at rice pudding temperature"; where the doctor arrived very nearly too late, where Walter was sent downstairs to boil unneeded water and the Irish setter pup Eh-la-bas! bounded in and onto my bed; where Dr. Rutherford said, "On the whole, I don't think we want that dog in here," grabbed him by the scruff and closed the door, washed his hands a second time and stood poised with his palms cupped to receive their burden, while the nurse instructed, "Pick a spot on the picture rail and aim the head for that."

So for decades I have thought of Tim's birth as a sad, slightly sour drama, and his little brother's as a comedy. For all I know, such moods and moments lie deep in the infant's consciousness. Perhaps they determine a worldview. Perhaps this notion is not some form of psychiatric hocus-pocus. It is certainly true that Tim was an earnest, honest child, more intent on justice than on fun—whereas Alex was a chatterbox, generous and inquisitive, given to wit and wordplay and irony. But doesn't that fit the pattern of first and second sons? Isn't it, anyway, largely a matter of genes and chance?

I can't now say how much or in what order information came in the few hours after Birgitt's call. Some things are preternaturally vivid in my memory; many are obliterated. I may have talked to her sister Ilke, her friend Rianne. I know that Birgitt was honest to the point of bluntness, even when it hurt her or me. I know that she blurted, "He did it in front of me! He did it in front of me!" And that I took this in with a doubleness others have described: I absolutely believed her and I also stood at a distance watching myself believe her, knowing it was all a mistake shortly to be explained. Tim was the most fiercely moral person I have ever known, responsible to the point of prudery, especially where family was concerned. *In front of me* made a picture I could see, but represented a vindictive force that was nothing to do with Tim. She said, "Neal was at the carnival. Thyra was asleep. She didn't even wake." I reacted with instant anger: *how could he do this to a*

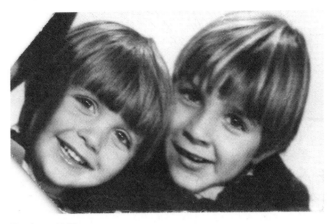

Brothers, 1969

three-and-a-half-year-old?! Birgitt asked me where he should be buried, and I remember that this seemed an offensive notion (*What? In the ground!?*) and at the same time considerate that she should ask my opinion. I had no doubt that he should lie in Namibia where he chose to live. I began to see that Peter and I must gird ourselves to go.

After we hung up, Peter and I huddled together. I said, "This is the big stuff." I don't know whether it struck me then that this was Army talk, throwaway; the thing Tim would have said.

"Yes, it is." He held me. We didn't sleep. We spent the next hours in that strange after-state of catastrophe, at once numb and intense, the body somehow silently thundering.

It was five o'clock when I called Alex to repeat the news. It was ten a.m. in London, not an unheard-of time to call, and he was ready with a narrative—his singing gig the night before, or the state of things at Piccadilly Station Underground. But he heard the strain of my response.

"What's wrong, Mom?"

"Honey, I have bad news. Tim has shot himself."

"Oh, my God. Is he dead?"

"Yes."

"Oh, my God. On purpose?"

"Yes."

"Oh, my God."

Unlike me he wept immediately, fully, blubberingly; and I sat in my vibrating space envying him that. I remembered, as I listened to him sob, the afternoon in Arizona when I had told the boys one by one that I had left their father. I climbed hand in hand with Tim up the bleachers of a baseball field behind my parents' house in Phoenix. It was the day after Christmas, Boxing Day to them. I told Tim we were not going back to England, and I tried haltingly to tell him why. Tim was nine, in some ways he was a nine-year-old man. He heard me out stoically. I admitted I was afraid of Walter, and he nodded: this was not news. His first question was "Will I ever see my dog again?" I said I didn't know, but I would try to get him back to England so he could. He asked, "Will I ever see Daddy again?" I said he would. He said, "We have to go tell Toby *right now*." And when we did, Tobyn Alexander burst into immediate, wailing sobs.

————

Tim was one of those boys for whom the paraphernalia of war held a fascination from toddlerhood. Guns, tanks, camouflage, planes—he learned commitment with model glue on the tip of a toothpick, and unlike most boys he never repudiated his first ambition. He spent three years in ROTC, four in the Army, and eight in the Reserve during which he volunteered for every available deployment: Germany, Bosnia, the Republic of Congo, Angola, Namibia. During this last assignment, 1998–99, he coordinated a project in mine removal from the embassy in Windhoek, clearing the detritus of the Namibian–Angolan war as a humanitarian gift of the United States. It was there that Tim met Birgitt. When his deployment ended, the Army decided no longer to staff his position, which would belong instead to the company that handled the field operation. So Tim came home to Florida and spent six months waiting for clearance to return to the same job as a civilian.

Strange how we accept the whims of a governmental monolith. It did not occur to me until more than a year after Tim's death that this small Pentagon decision, to privatize an Army staff position in mine removal, was part of a vast and pervasive policy. By the time Tim reached Iraq in 2003, half the jobs that had been done by soldiers from World War I to the first Gulf War would be farmed out to multinational corporations and their hired hands. From potato peeling to security, truck driving to engineering to mine removal to medicine, half the personnel in Afghanistan and Iraq would be civilians doing jobs that had always heretofore been done by the military. This is how the U.S. got by with an all-volunteer armed force: the grunt work and the specialized operations would be extracurricular. Of course, to get civilians to do war-zone jobs, the administration would have to pay. But Defense Secretary Donald Rumsfeld's theory was: quick-in, quick-out. An all-fighting force would make for near-immediate victory, and occupation would never be required. The corporations would make quick profits. The temp help could be cut loose without V.A. medical rights or a G.I Bill. The Pentagon need not keep track of their casualties.

In 1999 I saw none of this, nor could I at my most apocalyptic have imagined Tim as a worker ant in a global migration

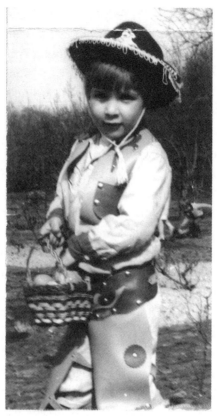

Cowboy; Sussex, England, 1968

from the public to the for-profit sphere. At the time it seemed to me good luck that Tim had a way to get back to the land-scape and the woman he had chosen. He and Birgitt married. A year later Thyra was born. Tim's company RONCO com-pleted the Namibian task, and he went on to head up a simi-lar program in Ethiopia. When that came to its end in the summer of '03, RONCO offered him, first, Washington, and then a project teaching mine removal to teams of Iraqis in the newly occupied Baghdad. Tim disliked Washington and hated desk jobs. He believed that the Iraq war was necessary, and after all his Army years as a "warrior without a war," he could barely contain his excitement at the prospect of going there. Of course, the family could not follow him to Iraq, so Tim and Birgitt made a pact: He would do one tour. If it was too dangerous, he would come home. Afterward they would go to Washington.

I was not afraid for him. I was adamantly against the war, but Tim and I had been on opposite political sides for most of his thirty-nine years, and we had learned to walk that minefield very well. I had written about it, and he had edited my mistakes in caliber, geography, and Army attitudes. Many of his beliefs made me uneasy still. Many of his enthusiasms were alien. But I accepted unease and alienation as part of the parental job description. Tim was committed to military values, and we were committed to each other, and when he told me he was heading for Iraq, I said, "You know how lucky I feel, don't you?—that you're taking mines out of the ground instead of putting them in. I know you'd put them in if that's what you were asked to do. I just think I lucked out you're doing this humanitarian thing." He laughed. "I know, Mom."

I was not afraid for him. It was early days in Iraq. The insurgency was still disorganized. Abductions had not begun in earnest. Abu Ghraib had not been heard from. And in any case I had long ago made peace with who Tim was. When, many years earlier, I faced his willingness to go to war, I thought it through: that if he should die in battle, *I* might think it was for nothing, but I would know he thought otherwise and would respect his choice. Wars happen because people try to make others live by their value systems. Families are rent for the same reason. I would not be a party to that. And Tim was broad-minded enough to say, "It's a good thing it's you who's the liberal, Mom. If I was the parent, I wouldn't let you be you the way you've let me be me."

———

He came to Tallahassee briefly in January 2004. He had been home to Namibia for Christmas and was returning to Baghdad by way of a de-mining conference in Tampa, with three days for a side trip to visit us. He came swinging down the airport carpet, as he had how many times before?—"Hi, Mom"—bearded, his hair thick and wavy, deeply tanned— "I look as Middle Eastern as I can"—energetic, opinionated, and enthused about the job. They were dealing with more unexploded American ordnance than mines, mainly cluster bombs, but all the same they were making progress, clearing land for farms, houses, soccer fields, and schools. He loved his men, whom he found, after the frustrations of Ethiopian officialdom, efficient and dedicated and quick to learn. They made him optimistic for an Iraqi democracy because, Sunni, Shiite, and Kurd, they worked together with mutual trust. His computer-full of photos gave me a sense of his life there: the low stucco building they had converted beside the 14th of July Bridge, the hands-linked march across the fields to mark the ordnance, the explosion that destroyed their find at the end of every day.

There was no sign of depression. On the contrary, Tim was slightly hyper. Since I'd been able to send only minimal Christmas presents to Africa, I gave him five hundred dollars to squander in the sales, and he came home flaunting his bargains. He sought out his best friend, John McBride, whom he'd known since fifth grade and for whom he'd been best man less than a year before. He said he was going back to Iraq for another six weeks only. He would be home in time for his fortieth birthday.

It was too hard to be away from Birgitt and Thyra—and even his stepson, Neal, who was becoming "a typical teenager, foul-mouthed and recalcitrant"—within, we divined, a more or less normal range. Peter and Tim bantered about whether boys or girls were more exasperating in the teen years.

But the second night it came out in a burst at table that he was disillusioned with the Bush administration and the Paul Bremer regime. Bitter at the failure to find the promised WMDs. Aghast that the entire Ba'athist structure had been dismantled, that his own company surcharged the government 60 percent on his salary, at the far more serious Halliburton graft, at the carelessness toward contractors' safety. He seethed: *the corruption, the incompetence, the lies, the greed, the stupidity!*

The truth is, I felt something very like joy, that he might be coming to recognize the flaws of capitalism, militarism, jingoism. I hadn't myself introduced a political topic for two years, not since a phone call a few days after 9/11 when he solemnly told me, "I think Bush is doing a magnificent job." That I hadn't challenged him then made me feel wise and cowardly by turns. Much later my brother Stan would say, "Tim was someone who thought that with ideals and a gun you could fix things," and I'd register how deep his disillusionment in Iraq must have cut. But at the time I was careful not to press. I didn't want him to hear I-told-you-so. So I squandered my one chance to ask what had in so short a time so changed his mind.

Later he held forth a little on the greed and graft in the government and in the country generally. He disparaged America's political dynasties and candidates in the pockets of big business, a system "inconsistent with democracy." We were happy to agree with him. Then he said that if he

were running things he would do away with "all unnecessary professions: sports stars, entertainers," and it took my
breath away, how little this was thought through. He meant
the celebrities who earn insane amounts of money—I had
no problem there—but "unnecessary professions"!? All the
struggling artists, inner-city coaches, underfunded theatres,
his mom as teacher of creative writing? Had he bought the
notion that some "Hollywood elite," rather than worship of
the bottom line, was responsible for our cultural schlock and
slime? I'm afraid I thought: *Unnecessary professions? Without
soldiers there would be no wars!* Yet I was proud of his work,
the unsoldiering work of mine removal, and of the cool courage he described as "warrior spirit," which led him to that
hard city to do that hard job.

———

Scraps of poetry pass through my mind that I love but haven't
understood till now. There's the Thomas Hardy lyric "Best
Times" that I memorized at nineteen, recounting a lifetime's
failure to recognize what's precious. It ends:

> *And that calm eve when you walked up the stair*
> *After a gaiety prolonged and rare,*
> *No thought soever*
> *That you might never*
> *Walk down again, struck me as I stood there.*

When I took, with my fancy new digital camera, the best
snapshot of Tim I'd ever taken; when we strolled down the
familiar airport corridor to put him on the plane; when he
gave me his hearty enveloping hug—hugs like handshakes
give you a measure of the person—no thought soever struck

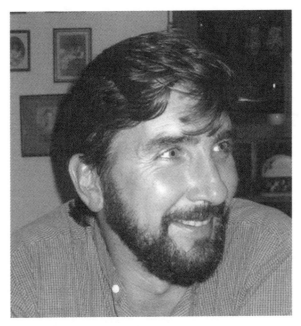

Tallahassee, Florida, January 2004

me. Tim hoisted his kit through the security barrier. Peter teased me that I had "fallen in love with him all over again." Like the retirees in a TV ad we agreed, laughing, that three days was about right for a visit from an offspring. Tim turned and waved. I was not afraid for him. In six weeks he would be home safe.

2.

There are reasons not to tell this story. Every serious biographer acknowledges that "a life" is in some way a cannibal enterprise. Mary Karr observed in *The New York Times* that "we memoirists occupy inherently muddy turf—cashing in on the misery of our loved ones and exploiting those who trust us." Tim is not *material*. I can distort and I can be misunderstood. When he died I wrote about him twice, shouts from the thick of pain and anger. One essay appeared under the headline "Tim's Last Kill," which seemed to attach me to the violence I wrote against. Two friends (both English) thought I exposed too much. One chilling email from a jihadist said, "Congratulations—that is great news!"

When, during his life, I wrote essays about Tim, it pleased him. He would grin and shine, proud of my being proud of him, and even of my being wry. But he was in himself reticent—markedly, sometimes admonishingly so. He was "hard to get to know." He specifically did not want his picture in the paper, and treated this as a given—something to do, I thought, with hugger-mugger ambition for Top Secret assignments.

More. Tim's tragedy is part of my story, but this is my story of his life and death. I'll draw, deliberately, conclusions I know he would reject. In the aftermath of divorce I considered suicide myself. If I had gone through with it, my parents might, with partial justification, have taken it to prove them right—about alcohol, cigarettes, "discretion" (which meant

14

sex), long hair and godlessness. I wouldn't have had a chance to edit, explain, rebut. No more will Tim.

Besides, it's been done before. William Styron definitively dealt with depression, Alfred Alvarez with suicide, Chris Hedges with the will to war. Joan Didion came to grips with grief so fast that she wrote a book within a year and published it before another year had ended. And that was a pure, clear cry, no one to blame and no mystery beyond mortality. Whereas Tim's death brought in its wake guilt and accusation and legal struggle and contradiction and regret and guess.

But I seem to have put a "2" in boldface at the top of this page, which means that I am writing a book. It's what I do. Peter says: "If you were a carpenter, you'd make a cabinet."

————

Not everyone deals with trauma by becoming manic, but many do, and I knew enough about myself to know this is my way. In the first days I became death's social secretary. Lists, calls, emails, letters, plane tickets to Africa. There were obituaries to write, music to find and fax for the funeral service in Namibia; poems to choose, photos to forward. People called and came. Family called and cried. Peter and I held each other but cried little. Thyra was told that her daddy had become a star, and she and I sang together on the phone: *Twinkle, Twinkle, Little Star.* I tracked down half-brothers and sisters, uncles who had fallen out of touch. I understood myself to be in a state of shock. I suspected from experience that I would pay for it later in emotional and perhaps bodily collapse; but beyond the fact that I could not stop, I also felt in some reassuring way that it *is* the way I cope, and must be trusted.

I had dealt with three deaths before: my father, my stepmother, and my father's sister Jessie. In each case I had experienced something like this hyper-efficiency. Together my brother Stan and I had parceled out the errands. We'd congratulated ourselves that we worked well together in a crisis. "Our folks raised nice kids," Stan said once, as a way of praising both our dad and us.

But those dead were all in their eighties or nineties and had been months or years in decline. There was urgency and distress (I once confronted an oncologist to tell him the chemo was too hard on Dad, so primed with my message that when he began, "I'm sorry; I have to stop treating your father. His heart can't take the chemotherapy"—I charged ahead and delivered my speech)—but we had lived with the expectation of these endings and could in each case speak of a *release*.

Tim's death was incomprehensible in a visceral way. I would look up from my desk, catch sight of a picture of him as a cherub in a Sussex garden, as a boy dangling a fishing pole over his father's lake in Minnesota, as a moustached soldier in his Army blues—and the unreality of the reality would register as liquid in my belly. *Dead? What is that?* I could see him swinging along the airport corridor, in through the kitchen door, "Hello the house!" It made no basic *sense* that this ordinary strand of the daily fabric could be un-knit.

And no mother ever prevented it by waiting up.

I was clear that there was to be no quarter given to shame. When my friend and colleague Jerry Stern suffered his long struggle with cancer, I'd been impressed that, whatever the doctors said, his friends could know it. I determined to emulate that openness. But it wasn't as easy as it seemed. Peter came home from his office at the university confessing that he'd mumbled "hunting accident" to two different colleagues. I told everyone that Tim had taken his own life, and how he was disillusioned by the war. But when it came to saying he had shot himself in front of his wife, I couldn't. I couldn't myself understand it. I had not forgiven it.

———

The flight from Tallahassee to Namibia is thirty hours. The leg from Atlanta to Johannesburg lasted seventeen, in one of those sardine-tin South African Airways planes nine seats across. Having booked at the last moment, we were in the center seats, Peter with too little room for his knees, his thighs bent awkwardly to the side. It was moment-by-moment. I tried to read Michael Chabon's *Werewolves in Their Youth* but found myself tracking again and again uncomprehendingly through the same beautifully formed sentence. I had in my mind the iconic Eddie Adams photo from Vietnam, of the Vietcong captive Bay Lop being shot in the head, how the blow of the bullet jerks his head sideways, so vivid that I remembered it in motion although it is a still. I saw Tim's head jerking sideways with the bullet's force, over and over and over. Again. Again. (It was family lore that as a toddler, when he wanted a game or story repeated, Tim would say, "Again. Another-gain.") A hundred times, a thousand, I saw the bullet coming from the side, Tim standing (he was not), the gun aimed at his temple from a little distance (it was not), his head jerking with the force. Again. I tried to distract myself with the movie *Sylvia*, which I watched squirming, moment-by-moment enduring, not because it was about suicide but because it devalued everything it depicted: the fifties, poetry, Plath's neurotic tempers, Hughes' eccentricity, their obsessive love. All made small.

I had one sleeping pill, and I took it, slept for perhaps four hours, a blessing, but woke to the Vietnam image, again, another-gain. In the airport at the Cape Town layover I eyed tchotchkes with trivial greed, wanting this lion key chain or that Herero doll. Souvenirs of Tim's country. Ashamed of this bizarre consumer impulse, I tried to quell it. Again. Again.

———

Namibia (pronounced *Nam-i-bee-ah*) is on the western coast of Africa, bounded by South Africa on the south, Angola on the north, and on the east Botswana, with which it shares the Kalahari Desert. The Caprivi Strip, a slender finger of land on the northern border, touches Zambia and meets Zimbabwe at Victoria Falls. "German South West Africa" was colonized toward the end of the 1800s—late, as the imperial carving up of Africa went, because of the formidable Namib Desert that formed an obstruction along the coast. Poor in farmland but rich in diamonds, it was invaded in World War I by South Africa, to whom the League of Nations awarded it after the war as a protectorate. When the League disbanded in 1946, a two-decade haggle began between the apartheid administration and the U.N., which eventually revoked the rights of South Africa and declared their occupation illegal. The South Africans were slow to go. At the same time several revolutionary groups had formed and fought, mainly in exile, to gain their independence. Of these the SWAPO (South West Africa People's Organization) eventually won power in the Republic of Namibia that formed in 1989. One anomaly of the long occupation is that English, spoken by about 7 percent of the populace, is still the official language. However, the German missionaries had done their work; the dominant religion among the total population, black and white, is Lutheran.

Namibia's landscape, as I had learned on our first visit there—in 1998, only a few weeks after Tim and Birgitt met—is strikingly like the Arizona of my childhood: the brown hills covered with gray-green scrub, the perpetual ring of far mountains, the black two-lane highway cutting straight to the horizon and shimmering with mirage. The difference is that across this plain, beside the road, you are likely to spot a rhino, a herd of springbok or elephants, a hyena, a trio of giraffes. April is autumn in the southern hemisphere, and Namibia on a latitude that would equate to Mexico's in the northern. The air is clear and warm. Tim used to call it "Africa Lite."

I had not seen Tim and Birgitt's house, which sits on a hill in the district of Windhoek called Eros, the plot surrounded by a security wall topped with razor wire. This chilling sight is standard for the white middle class of Namibia, where violent crime is less than in America but thievery and vandalism rife. Within the wall a very steep drive leads up to a ranch one-story, laid out with bedrooms at one end, kitchen and living-dining in the middle, and up a few steps a rec room leading out onto a veranda. The view (Arizona again) is far desert and mountain over the massed walls of the houses.

Tim's family were waiting for us: Birgitt who is third-generation Namibian of German and Afrikaans descent, slender and tall, her pretty features well-defined, her chin pert and determined under soft red-brown hair; Neal, who might at fourteen pose for a model of the blond Aryan; and 3-year-old Thyra, Tim's only child and my youngest granddaughter, also brightly blond, her hair cut in a *gamine* shag, her eyes blue but grayer than Tim's. A photo of her laid next to one of Tim at the same age might be of his twin.

Birgitt wanted urgently to walk me at once through what happened, and though I was exhausted and felt brutalized by the scene, I also wanted this. I wanted to be brutalized, to cut through my zombie state. Birgitt's friend Rianne Selle had tactfully rearranged the furniture so that dining and living rooms had changed place, which meant I sat on the couch where the dining table was before, while Birgitt described to me how Tim killed himself in that same space.

Tim's friend and hunting companion Pieter had brought him home on the Friday morning from a game farm; he had entered here. And here he had stood, his face red and swollen so that she had asked him what was wrong. Had he been partying? No, he hadn't slept. The trip was a disaster. He had not wanted to go for a cull, had not wanted to shoot at night, with Pieter's gun, from a moving vehicle. He had wounded a gemsbok (or oryx, a kind of antelope) and they had not been able to track it, meaning it had wandered off to die in pain. He could not get over it. She said, "But there are three people here who love you, so please let your buck go." He could not. Everything had gone wrong. The buck, danger for his men in Iraq, a rifle maker who had ripped him off. Birgitt asked, "And us?" and he, by the kitchen here, so that Martha, their young housekeeper, had seen it, had put his arms around her, "No, not us."

In the bedroom along that hall he had tried to put Thyra down for her nap, but she'd screamed for her mother, and he slammed the door. Here in the living room in the afternoon he had quarreled with Neal, who wanted to go to the carnival with friends. Tim considered these boys a bad influence, too old for Neal, likely to be into drugs. That quarrel resolved, he had driven Neal to the carnival himself, had come back here, to the dining room, with take-out supper, after which he and Birgitt began a game of cards.

He put Thyra to bed. It took an unusually long time, and when he returned he put his head in his hands. "That was so difficult."

She thought him too tired, but he said they should finish their game. At some point he said, "I'm tired of being the bad man."

She said, "Honey, you're not the bad man. It's only when you're down you feel that way."

He swept his arm in the air. "I hate Neal!"

"What?!"

And immediately, "I didn't mean it. I take it back." He jabbed his finger toward her. "But you'd better get me some help!"

Irritated, she replied, "Yes, I will, because I'm sick and tired of cheering you up all the time."

She went to the kitchen, through that door. He went, it seemed, to the bedroom, down that hall. And when they were back at the table, her attention on shuffling the cards, he said: "Is that what you've been doing for the last five years, cheering me up?" And, sitting, the barrel of the gun on the maxilla just below his right temple, he tucked his face toward his right shoulder, squinted hard (she demonstrated this clench-faced look), pulled the trigger, aiming upward so that the bullet came out the upper left cranium and went through the black-and-beige drapes (she poked a finger through the hole) over a long horizontal window. Here was the jagged hole in the glass.

Her first reaction was fury. She screamed, "Coward!" and ran to telephone her brother Jacques, but as luck would have it the phone was dead. She fumbled trying to find her cell, found it, called Jacques, then Ilke and Rianne. Only then did it occur to her to push the security button that would bring the police.

Tim had fallen to the floor on his side, just here, the gun concealed under him. She had not heard the shot, but she saw a "thumbed-sized" piece of his brain on the floor. She thought he sighed. She thought: *They can fix him. They can put him back together.*

Jacques came immediately and—deciding Tim was still breathing—*carried* his dead weight (how? down that 45-angle drive!) to his car. The hospital is right around the corner, but Jacques overshot it, had to turn around, and when he stopped took Tim's face in his hands. "Do you want to live this way, Tim?"

It isn't clear whether Tim was then alive. Most probably not. Most probably, what they took for breathing was the chemical reaction that used to be thought of as the soul taking leave. The doctor said that in any case it was better that he died; he'd have been without speech, without movement. This struck me as both true—Tim in that state would have wanted to kill himself again—and also what you say at the vet's office of a damaged dog. Three months later I wrote these events in my journal with ice still in my fingers.

Sometime later that night, as they tried to call us, Rianne and Ilke mopped the blood from the carpet. A professional cleaner had improved the job before Peter and I arrived. There was a skin from a slaughtered zebra at my feet, masking the spot.

———

Friends and family flowed in and out of the house or crowded around a long table on the veranda—gentle Ilke and doe-eyed Rianne, Birgitt's half-brother Jacques and cousin Jean Paul and his mother Lin, Neal's grandmother Marienne, friends Hannelore, Volker, Robert, and Laura; and Martha, who arrived every day to clean up, weeping, after us all.

Birgitt and I on the other hand were deranged. We shared an overarching sense that what had happened to Tim was incomprehensible, and that we would see the aftermath through. Nevertheless, horrific and ludicrous suspicions spilled from both of us.

That first afternoon Birgitt asked why Tim was so determined that Neal should not go to Carnival. "Why *so* angry? It makes you wonder if he thought, if he did all of us, no one would suffer."

I did not understand what she meant. "If he what?"

"Was he going to kill all of us?"

I said, "I can't hear this. I'm sorry." I had not yet had any rest. I went to the spare room that had been assigned. Birgitt followed and sat on the bed. She asked if she'd been too rough for me, something to that effect. I said yes, I could not entertain what she suggested. She left. I may have slept a little, maybe not.

The next morning the police arrived, and it was my turn for fantasy. What suspicions did they entertain? What evidence did they hold? They questioned Birgitt for two hours. When they left she said, "The case is not closed." My heart stuttered at this, but she shrugged. "Well, how does it look?" They had tested her hands for powder burns the night of Tim's death, and she'd cried, "Here! Handcuff me! Put me in the electric chair right now!"

Food appeared. Drinks. Lasagne. Talk on the veranda. Ilke and I worked on the funeral program against some untimely computer glitch. Alex arrived from England and in his enveloping hug (so like Tim's!) I was able to cry a little. Taller than his brother, heavier and more expansive, Alex entered any gathering including this one at a stride. Where his brother would have stood for a time on the sidelines, reconnoitering, Alex was instantly gregarious, his voice an instrument of power. (Why was he the pacifist, Tim the warrior?)

Children ran in and out. I read to Thyra. I was no

longer efficient, but blank and clumsy. Once, catching sight
of Neal crossing to his room deep in thought, there came
unbidden a memory of Tim not much younger, after he had
seen some vampire movie. It was hot in his attic bedroom,
but he wanted the windows closed. He sheepishly assured
me he knew vampires weren't real, and I said, "No, but the
fear is real. We'll close the windows to keep out the fear."
Why had I had no such wisdom for him now, here, when
the need was pressing?

Thursday morning the preacher came, a hugely tall, pit-
ted-faced man named Trauernicht (which means literally *don't
mourn*). He was consoling in a preacherly way, but when I
said that I wanted to read a poem at Tim's funeral, he assured
me that it would be too difficult. No, I said, I wanted to, and
I could. I held on to this scrap of what appeared to represent
"normality." I had stood up for my father and his sister and I
would do so for Tim.

Birgitt wove a litany through the day: "Tim was *not*
depressed! He was fine! He was joking around with friends!"
The topic turned to depression, how well it could be hidden,
and someone said, "Any thinking person has considered suicide." Birgitt said, "Not I!" We stood in that kitchen where
Tim had stood, a dozen who were known to him but not to
me, drinks in hand, conversationally establishing that only
two of us could say we had not given serious thought to taking our own lives.

It was disorienting to move between these plaster walls,
among shabby and eclectic furniture ("We were moving; it
wasn't worth buying new"). I had visited Tim in Gainesville,
Hawaii, Tallahassee, Windhoek. I had always made a point of
wanting to see where he sat as we talked on the phone, where
he worked on the computer, where he whipped up enchiladas

or shrimp scampi. It made him real, I said. Now, in this space I had never seen and to which he would never return, he was doubly absent. Alex sat on the veranda drinking local beer, chatting in wide-ranging conversation with the friends Tim would never see again. Images of his life momently materialized and slipped into past tense, like film footage of an actor in an obituary.

That is, if Birgitt's grieving took the form of lashing out, mine took the form of random anxiety. Later in bed Peter held me while I trembled, and did not try to contradict my fear. Awake again at five, I went to look out the window, spread back the curtain, and a six-inch cricket or katydid leapt at my hand. I screamed. Peter woke and killed it, calmed me again, stroked my hair and wrapped himself around me.

"We have to get through five days. We have to do it, and we can."

Next morning Rianne took Peter, Alex, and me to town, herded us from store to store to buy shoes for Thyra, for me a pair of horn earrings with pale stars in them, (*Twinkle, Twinkle, Little Star*), and the trinkets I had denied myself in Cape Town. The shopping was genuine distraction. I felt no guilt, just a further dislocation, time out of time.

———

Friday, April 30; a full week since his death. The police had only now released Tim's body. Birgitt and Neal, Peter, Alex, and I felt we must see him. I was unprepared and did not realize I was unprepared, I think because all the dead I have seen, though some were dear to me, have been old people in tufted satin, discreetly decorated by the embalmer's art.

But this was a police station on the outskirts of Windhoek: dry desert and a shed-like building covered in scrofulous plaster. The plain box coffin was behind a window slanted so that you looked down through it, and Tim was covered to the neck by a rumpled sheet, his wide-brim Australian hunting hat shoved down as if to hide, though it did not, an indentation in his forehead like the meeting of three ravines. This was not the site of his wound and I know no explanation for it. Crude makeup on his jaw did not conceal that the skin was bruised. On the bridge of his nose was a bright red spot at exactly the point where he had broken it twenty years ago in an ROTC "war game." He was vividly recognizable but death was also recognizable. He did not look peaceful. He did not look asleep. I felt faint and, simultaneously, that it was necessary I had come. Alex pulled my arm over his shoulder to support me. Peter put a hand under my other arm, and we made our way out. It had taken perhaps two minutes.

This image of my dead son is "seared into my memory," which idiom aptly suggests the sound and pain of a branding iron. Weeks later, on a train through the Sussex landscape of Tim's childhood, it came to me that of the many dozens of images I have of Tim, all are alive but this one breathtaking negative of all the others. Dozens of mental pictures, animated and changing second by second—splashing in his baby bath, coasting on his first bicycle down the drive, dropping his parachuted Action Man over the balcony, playing soldier in the Tallahassee pines, speed-skating, dismantling the motor of his MG, peeling apples, driving me over the mountains of Oahu, making thyme gravy for Thanksgiving, swinging in the kitchen door, "Hi, Momma," "Love you, Mom"—and only the one image in stasis, brief, eternal.

3.

Shock is the psyche's Novocaine. One brutal jab and the pain is blocked by partial paralysis. Later I would have time to ponder *never* and *if only*. There would be nights to consider the cruelty of *in the ground*. In Windhoek for the moment I only knew that parts of me didn't work. My arms disposed themselves at inconvenient angles. My face, I think, was set in a look of ingratiating reasonableness, as of someone who didn't want to get too much in the way. Compassion all around me took the form of incredulity—*Not Tim!* But for myself, instead of anguish or disbelief, I felt a hollow humming, little eruptions of alarm or guilt. My mind fastened on half-sentences of which the completing clause wafted ceilingward.

May Day 2003 George Bush had declared the Mission Accomplished. May Day 2004 we readied ourselves to bury Tim. We bathed and dressed. I used my curling iron to turn under my stubbornly straight hair. Peter hovered. Alex dressed in full McKenzie kilt, struggling with the complicated garters and tie, to honor his brother, who had been proud of their Scottish heritage. A striking black couple arrived, he in severely western suit and tie, she in a traditional Herero gown of patterned white silk and matching headdress. I wore a black shift with a burned-velvet blouse, of which a friend had observed that it had a ghostly quality, "there and not there." Bright Thyra, in the black-with-roses velvet dress I had made her for Christmas, the new silver shoes, asked where we were going, and I said we were going to a ceremony for Daddy. She took up this word and used it several times, as if placing the occasion in her mind.

————

The Windhoek mortuary is a low modern building in a pleasant setting of fan-shaped trees and lawns and flowers. Inside there was a wooden structure of some kind that I mentally addressed as the coffin before I recognized the hardwood box a little to the left of it, that last snapshot I had taken of him in January propped in front. My failure of focus seems odd and apt, a little comic. Trauernicht was not. He was unexpectedly and inappropriately fulsome in his piety. Later I could not remember whether Trauernicht preached in English or German, although, of the little I could take in that day, I could understand how often we were assured that *Jesus the Redeemer* would *redeem*. Trauernicht's tone conveyed he was embarrassed by suicide and assumed we were as well. "*Ach Bleib mit Deiner Gnade bei uns, Herr Jesu Christ*" we irrelevantly sang ("Maintain your love for us, Lord Jesus"), and then the "Battle Hymn of the Republic"—a further oxymoron as far as I was concerned, though Tim would have approved. "Amazing Grace" is a lovely song; so what? This was a funeral like other funerals, and therefore little to do with Tim. *Dead? What is that?*

Ten years before, a friend had offered, for the memorial service of another friend, a poem by Randall Jarrell patterned after Rilke, and it had become precious to me, and I read it, tears rolling but not in my throat, not such that I couldn't be understood.

> *If I could I would sing you to sleep.*
> *I would give you my hand to keep*

In yours till you fell asleep,
And take it away then, slowly.
I would sit by you and be...

The reading of this poem was the only time during that service I felt connected to Tim, but afterward it was the images of others, of tenderness and comedy, that stayed with and to an extent consoled me. Alex in his kilt, Peter in unaccustomed jacket and tie, Neal, and three others carried the coffin down the aisle and into a white van. Alex later recalled how light the coffin seemed, and how the line "He ain't heavy, he's my brother" sang inanely in his head. Behind the van, he marched in the fore, one foot after another, a military bearing. Thyra walked beside me and we sang "Twinkle, Twinkle, Little Star." Ilke handed out long-stemmed roses from a bucket, and Thyra asked what they were for. I said, "We're going to plant the roses for Daddy." She accepted this.

It was better to be outside in the warm air. We made our slow way to the gravesite, passing through a crowd of perhaps a hundred Herero waiting for their cortège, the women in satin full-skirted dresses and matching headdresses shaped to mimic long-horned cattle, staring in amaze at Alex in his kilt regalia as he dirge-marched behind the coffin.

The coffin was lowered and we passed, tossing the roses in. Thyra stood, sun on her platinum hair and silver shoes, spooning little spadesful of sand onto the flowers. Trauernicht began to drone again. The Herero, having arrived by now, brought a funeral-jazzy band that all but drowned him out. I caught Alex's eye; we nodded: *yes, add Walter to the mix*—the boys' father, who was a great lover of New Orleans jazz.

Later Thyra told me that "the ceremony was very long and very hot, but very beautiful."

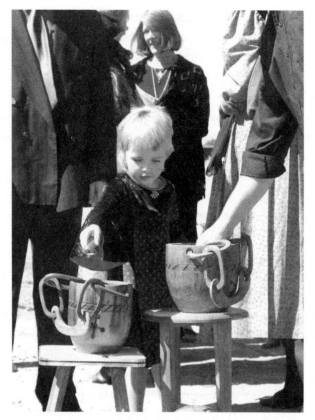

Thyra "planting the roses," Windhoek, Namibia, May 1st 2004.

After the lunch crowds had come and gone, Birgitt was eager to take us to the hill site where she and Tim had married. I think now that this was a nostalgic impulse on her part, but in my disconnected state I put a paranoid spin on it.

In 1999, Birgitt and Tim had been romantically intent on being married on millennium eve. As Peter and I were to spend that Christmas in London visiting Alex, they proposed and supposed we would fly down for it. It's hard at this point to recapture the doomsday scenario that surrounded Y2K (and about which Tim was in any case dismissive), but I was nervous about boarding in the first days of the new millennium a South African Airways plane for a fourteen-hour flight back to London. I thought they could change the date to one that was more comfortable for us. Tim shrugged off my fears and thought I should overcome them. We never quarreled about it, and I spent a good part of the London holidays finding and shipping him the perfect tux. But our failure to make their wedding had no doubt festered. Later, when they were in Tallahassee, Tim had pressed us to come for a visit.

I said, "You know, I'm in my sixties. I can't make a thirty-hour flight for a ten-day holiday."

Tim said flippantly, "Then stay two weeks."

I said, "I can't do it, Tim. I'm serious."

He sobered. "I didn't know that, Mom."

"I'll come to visit you from London, when I've adjusted to the jet lag, but not from Florida. I'm too old."

I was aware of the irony, that I was now in Namibia for a five-day stay of zero holiday content; and also that this tender area of in-law relations had prompted Birgitt to complain that Tim thought we preferred the London family. But I spell this out in logical sequence now, whereas on the afternoon of Tim's funeral I was lunatic.

We set out, the four of us—Birgitt, Peter, Alex and me—away from Windhoek across the scrub-covered hills. There was a road, and then a trail, and then a maze of tracks barely visible through the grass, which petered out while Birgitt said, "Oh, that's not it, we need to go back to the last turn," or "Maybe it's off of that road," and, "Don't worry, we'll find it."

But we got farther and farther into the hills, lacking vantage point or even a sense of where the sun would set—which it would do, was doing, the light diminishing and yellowing. The turns got more confusing and I became first worried that we would be stuck here for the night (How cold? How dark? What animals?)—and then, for a moment of uncontrollable panic, that Birgitt meant to abandon us. After forty-five minutes of this tortuous winding, she stopped the car. "This is it." We got out and climbed the last quarter mile.

With no more to fear, of course, than a beautiful plateau on a hilltop, a view of the sunset behind a handsome tree. From her bag Birgitt produced stemmed glasses; Alex brought out a bottle of cognac. We toasted Tim.

———

Behavior carries you. When your condition is no longer exactly shock, but a gingerly testing of the reality, habit still impels you forward, making little folds in time. I never didn't know how to put on my underwear, slacks, shoes. I knew the napkin went in my lap, the tines of the fork would lift the meat. If no food appeared I knew how to look in the fridge, grate cheese, and fold an omelet over. Then, staring into the pan I might abruptly think: *You can't make an omelet without breaking eggs.* Or my mind would offer: *All the king's horses and all the king's men . . .* The raw skin at the edge of the wound would lift. Nevertheless I could steady myself on the counter, put the dishes on the table, say at large: *Come on, everybody, you must eat.*

When strangers opened their arms, I appropriately walked into them. Sometimes I would think enviously of Eastern women covering their faces with black cloth, keening like ambulance sirens, flinging themselves prostrate on the floor.

And then it would occur to me that the opposite must also happen: that while a Muslim mourner performs her histrionic ritual of grief, she must sometimes wish she could just sag, dumb, into a stranger's hug.

———

Meanwhile information came as mismatched fragments, some suggesting a coherent picture, some not at all. I learned from Birgitt that as long ago as November—Tim would not have told me this—the de-mining team rode with an Army security convoy that had fired live bullets into Iraqi houses. "And now," Tim told her, "they deny it was civilians." She asked him why. With disgust: "So they don't have to pay compensation."

I learned the full extent of his quarrel with RONCO at the conference in Tampa after he left Tallahassee. The company had announced its intention to forbid the team to carry weapons. Tim said in that case he would quit. He said bitterly that RONCO was more concerned with lawsuits than the men's lives. In the green zone, he'd taken to collecting the weapons after hours, handing them out in the morning. He slept in an armory.

I learned that on his last flight out of Baghdad his plane had given off shafts of light, and Tim thought they were under missile attack. He was terrified. "There was nothing I could do. I thought I'd come this far only to die on the way out." Weeks later, only days before he died, he was repairing a roof no more than ten feet from the ground, and when he ascended, the ladder shook so badly that the builder asked if he was afraid of heights. Tim was a paratrooper. He loved nothing more than jumping out of planes.

When he left Iraq his men had given him a gilded statue

of a rearing horse, to honor him, they said, for being their "workhorse." The front leg had broken off en route. Back home in Namibia Tim tried and failed to glue it back on, and Birgitt thought he had taken this failure as a symbol.

Some of his friends said he'd been "perfectly normal" or "congenial, as always." But one acquaintance judged him "too cool, too relaxed for someone just out of a war zone," and another observed he couldn't tolerate noise, especially children's noise. Sometimes he seemed abstracted and far away. Some noticed that he wouldn't talk about Iraq, and to one he said, "You don't live there. You just survive." Thyra's teacher, though, had told Birgitt that the love between father and daughter shone out between them, and that Tim "had a sunshine personality."

Rianne thought the same, and was taken aback when Tim carped to her in trivial ways—about Birgitt's cooking, her weight, that she "always took Neal's side." He threatened that he would go back to the States, then to another friend said he would not go to Washington: "It isn't going to happen." To Birgitt he declared that he would not go to England to visit the family.

He was drinking more. He didn't sleep. Sometimes he was petulant and clingy; another time he drove back from the beach fast enough to scare her and the children. He told Birgitt (in Army argot) that he was always aroused at night. He said, "Something's wrong. I'm down."

After the Madrid bombing and the strafing of Fallujah, he'd become a news junkie, which he never was before. To one friend he said, "I should go back," but to another, speaking of the occupation, "There is murder and killing going on that should not be" and to a third, "I'm ashamed to be an American."

On the day of his death, unprecedentedly, Tim watched cartoons with Thyra for more than two hours. On the trip to the carnival that afternoon, Neal asked him, "What's wrong with you today?" and Tim said, "It's always difficult for me this time of year." No one could figure out what he'd meant by that. Tim told Neal and only Neal that his rifle bullet had hit the gemsbok in the face—he knew this because they'd found a tooth.

The night he died he left the bedroom floor strewn with bullets. There was a single round in the clip. What did that mean? And why would his hunting buddy and best friend Pieter not come to the funeral?

A few of these scraps I'd had from Tim, by phone or email when he was in Iraq or after. Some I heard in Namibia after his death, or later still. Many contradicted others. There was not in early May of 2004 any body of evidence as would emerge toward the end of that year, of erratic anger, marital discord, and the suicide rate of Iraq survivors. The Army study had not been released that showed a one-in-three rate of depression and anxiety for Iraq veterans. The statistical incidence of post-Iraq post-traumatic stress disorder had not been calculated. Cindy Sheehan had not camped out in Crawford, Texas. *Doonesbury's* "B.D." had not begun to treat his family to drunken rants. Colonel Ted Westhusing had not been found shot dead in his trailer on a Baghdad base, nor e-mailed his family that honor had been replaced by profit. He had not yet written: "I am sullied. I came to serve honorably and feel dishonored."

———

The morning after the funeral, descending the few steps from the TV room, I slipped and fell spread-eagle across the carpet where Tim had fallen. I lay there, in no hurry to rise, letting myself sink cheek-to-floor beside the zebra skin. I felt the prickling of the fibers against my face. My breath caught warm in the woolen nap. I welcomed the sting of a scrape on my knee where I had torn a hole in my cropped pants.

Near that spot, too, Birgitt had placed three dozen deep-red roses, Tim's usual choice for her. A couple of hours after I fell, Neal knocked over the vase and so poured half a gallon of water on the spot where his blood had been.

——

On the plane home I didn't try to read or watch a movie, but penned, furiously, a "letter to the NRA." I also sketched out a children's book, *My Daddy Was a Star*, but I never finished it. I couldn't get the plotting right. Did the stars somehow need him, or did he choose them of his own free will? In preference to his family?

No comfort there.

4.

Back from Namibia, Peter asked what film we'd seen the night of Tim's death. I didn't know. He found the ticket stubs in his pocket. The movie was called *Intermission*. We looked it up on the Internet. There displayed for us were the stars, the plot, the reviews, and an album of stills. We did not recognize any of them. It was total memory-wipe, as if we'd waked in a hospital after an accident.

Memories luminous and stark appeared in every square foot of the house. I wandered through to exercise, not exorcize, them, acknowledging Tim's "ghost." He was in the open door flicking his cigarette out over the azalea bushes. He was in shirtsleeves at the stove, in a suit and ascot next to the stairs; a brown-legged kid climbing the porch pole, a comical teen blow-drying his hair in the attic mirror, a bearded techie fixing the hard drive in my study. Here in the linen cupboard was the tree-printed sheet set he picked for the waterbed of his youth, shabby but serviceable still. Back in the kitchen was a tumbler he used to take out to the pool time after time because it was the biggest glass we had. Time after time I *tsked* under my breath, not wanting to pick those shards out of the mulch.

How could I bear it that he was broken and the glass intact?

———

Violent, too-early death surfaced in the stories of every family we knew. Bessie's son died in an accident, as did Lou's sister, Randy's mom. Beth lost a father, Hilda a mother and brother,

37

Stuart a son to suicide. When we looked at our own (middle-class, law-abiding, decent, mostly church-going) families, the toll was high: Peter's grandfather had accidentally shot the teenage son of a friend on a hunting trip, had never recovered from the guilt and had eventually taken his own life. Peter's nephew and namesake, an addict, had hanged himself only two years before. Tim's paternal grandfather, racked by his mistress's death and financial crisis, had ended his own life by gassing himself. Tim's cousin Yannick had died in a fall that may or may not have been his choice, so that when I spoke to his father, Tim's uncle Hans, he cried in anguish, "What's wrong with the Eysselincks?"

That suicidal behavior runs in families is a statistical fact, though the augmented risk is still no more than two in a thousand. For no precisely understood reason, suicidal behavior tends to skip a generation. Girls are less likely than boys to take their lives. Scientists disagree on whether there is a "suicide gene" or only inherited traits such as impetuosity, bipolarity, or addiction. It's clear that the serotonin system is involved and that this system is intricately interactive with neurobiology, childhood experience, and mental health.

Did I think of Tim's grandfather's suicide as relevant to the boys? Yes and no. It was a dramatic fact and factor in Walter's life, and made him contemptuous of mental illness. But I was well aware of the mortal danger of car accidents, and I regularly put the boys in the car. Statistically my impulse was right, that the road was the greater risk.

Now the dead children and the suicides magically proliferated on TV. This cop, that horror show, this "in-depth" coverage, that disaster trash. *CSI: Miami* swings between clinical gore and saccharine kids. Philip Seymour Hoffman in *Empire Falls* stands movingly, memorably, in a gazebo with a pistol at his head. *Law & Order* "rips from the headlines" perhaps one child in half a dozen murders. Watching television I pointed these out to Peter almost daily: *dead child, dead child.* I found that I could perfectly well take violent death on the large or small screen as long as it had what we used to call "redeeming social value"; as long as it dealt seriously with the human struggle. The casual, technically competent gore that hourly spilled from the tube sent me out of the room.

I have, as a matter of literary course, dealt in fictional death myself. In one novel a politician owes his election to the murder of his daughter; in another a girl spurs her horse over the edge of a marble quarry when she discovers her father *in delicto*; in yet another an actress is accidentally strangled. At least four heroines consider suicide but choose life. There's a Cassandra figure who bizarrely claims, "Everyone loses a child." I've even done a surreal *Medea.* The point of my play is that we need the ordering force of words in order to accept the unacceptable. My "Media" says, "This is my story. If I had some other story, then who would I be?"

I remembered that in the few months after Tim was born—a colicky, fretful child—there were moments when I felt, *I'll never have any identity again except as Tim's mother.* It took me a while to reemerge as a person in my own right, saying: *I am* also *Tim's mother.*

Now, henceforth, I am to be the mother of a suicide. *Also*, to be sure. But forever and always also that.

If I had some other story, then who would I be?

When I was depressed and traumatized by leaving my marriage, in Illinois in 1972, I saw a therapist, first name Polly, last name lost, whom I told that I had thoughts of suicide. She said that was okay, I had a right to act on them, as long as I waited until my parents were both dead and my youngest child was eighteen. I remember thinking that if I could live that long there was no point killing myself at all; and that my suicide might of course harm my children (would their father take proper care of them?—I had scant notion of how loss itself might skew their lives); but that it had scarcely anything at all to do with my parents, who would, yes, be shocked, but when had they not been shocked at my life? They could have so little understanding of my pain that I hardly had any obligation to live for their sakes. When I remember that younger self, I cannot suppose Tim had any space in his tortured psyche to spare for me.

——

I read Judy Collins's touching memoir of her son who took his life, *Sanity and Grace*, William Styron's *Darkness Visible*, Edwin Shneidman's *Autopsy of a Suicide,* John Miller's anthology of great writers *On Suicide*. I re-read A. Alvarez's *The Savage God*. Both James Hillman, in *Suicide and the Soul,* and David Hume, in *On Suicide,* take on the common, harsh belief that suicide is a sin against the self, society, and/or God. Hillman traces the condemnation through human institutions; Hume puts his energy into justifying individual choice. "I believe that no man ever threw away his life while it was worth keeping." Gingerly I test this against what I know of Tim's life. I weigh it on one hand, and on the other, "Suicide is a permanent solution to a temporary problem." Is it only because I'm his mother that the latter has the clearer ring of truth?

I remember the feeling of the moment of decision before a violent act. Once I threw a flower pot at a wall. Once to get Walter's attention I deliberately turned a car over into a ditch. Several times I picked up my keys, walked out and drove away. I have always been, oddly perhaps, interested in the charged pause before such an act. One of my characters styles it, "The calm before the storm. That second of hesitation before the donor bends to sign. The moment the diver bounces from the board and hangs outstretched. Michael Jordan treading air. Baryshnikov in flight." What was in Tim's mind between the moment he said, "Is that what you've been doing...?" and the second he retracted the muscles of his trigger finger. And after that? Tad Friend records that Golden Gate jumpers who survive "often regret their decision in mid-air." Tobias Wolff, in "Bullet in the Brain" traces (by omission, mainly: no thought of parents, wife, or child; no memory of joy in his profession) the last synapses of a dying man. Bob Butler in *Severance* imagines the precisely calculated 240 last words, a minute and half, of the thoughts of historical victims of decapitation. Did Tim have time, too late, to change his mind? Waking early in the months after his death I would think these thoughts for him: *I take it back; I didn't mean it; I want my life,* and then, backing up to the moment of hesitation, I mother-talked him out of it: *please don't, sweetheart; think again; whatever it is, we can find and fix it...*

No comfort there.

———

Now no memory of him could surface without the clenching in my stomach that meant: *he's gone.*

This: He was in a baby buggy someone had given us, an expensive shiny thing, parked in my study in Ghent where he was born. I had picked a fistful of lilies of the valley and stuck them between two chrome bars on the buggy frame. He—fat, gurgling, three or four months old, in pale blue wool pants like baby lederhosen—flung his arms about at random and happened to hit the flowers. Which bounced. This happened

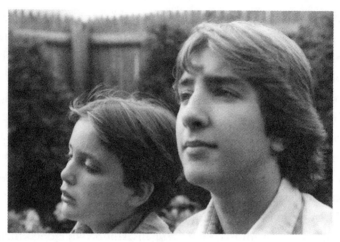

The brothers Toby & Tim, Tallahassee, c. 1976

three or four times and then, as I watched, he figured it out. That it was part of himself that made the white thing move. There was *concentration* on his face. He aimed his arm. It worked. Again. Not in full control but trying, doing. I felt privileged to have seen the moment.

I have thought of, probably told, this incident many times. But now it no longer exists on a continuum of discovery, capacity, control. It was a moment that meant a future. And now does not.

Or this: Soon after we moved into the house on De Soto Street—the boys would have been nine and twelve—Alex put a ball through a mullioned pane in a neighbor's porch door. I called a glazier and then called the boys together, sat them down. "Everyone is allowed one window," I said. "After that, if you break another you have to work to pay it off."

So far so good. The repair cost $25 and Alex never broke another. When Tim destroyed his *one*, though, it was a $400 plate glass skylight set oblique into a mansion roof. He'd put a BB through it with his birthday present. I went to confront and apologize to the owner. She turned out to be a widow in her late fifties, corpulent, in dowager mode. She presented the hole in her skylight—the exact size of a BB, an inch from the frame—which needed a squint to see and could have been plugged with a drop of glue. Four hundred dollars was most of a biweekly paycheck for me, but it was not my call. The widow and I made small talk while I wrote the check. I suppose I was chattering about children, the scrapes they get into, the trouble they cause—because she crossed the room to bring me a framed 8x10 photo of a teenage girl: her daughter, who had died of leukemia some ten years before. The widow began to tell stories compulsively, as I'm doing now. She eulogized the lost girl, her beauty, her intelligence, her perfect manners. She went through the stages of the disease, the Latinate terms, and the decline, intense. She cried softly. I felt both touched and awkward, honored and imposed upon. The recitation went on and on. After some time I reached out a hand to comfort her. I touched her arm. She drew up, startled, coldly took the check, and showed me out.

I have tried several times to write about this, but I found I never knew the point. It was an afternoon of small turns of gathering emotion, but meaning what, and to what end? Now I must notice, which I never did before, that the anecdote begins with a gun that I gave Tim—I suppose the last in a series of plastic blasters, water pistols, stick-wood rifles and battery-operated lasers. I had pacifist friends who wouldn't give a little boy a gun, but that was too pious for me. *They'll just point their fingers*, I said. *They'll just whittle twigs.*

Alvarez says of the suicide that "no one is promiscuous in his way of dying. A man who has decided to hang himself will never jump in front of a train."

———

A dear friend, slightly flaky, with a 24-karat heart, asked us to a dinner party. In the course of the table chat, she told a funny story about her brother and a cowboy gun, a Colt or some such Old West familiar. She said, "And I have the gun!"—which she proceeded to produce from a whatnot cabinet. She passed it around the table. "Feel how heavy it is!" I did not want to touch it. As it came 'round I pushed my chair back as discreetly as I might and excused myself to the bathroom, where I splashed my face and washed my hands.

When I came out she waylaid me in the living room. "Oh, Janet! I'm so sorry. I knew that would happen to you. But I *didn't* want it to be me that did it. I'm *so* sorry." I demurred, agreed that it was bound to happen; not to worry. "*Mea culpa!*" she insisted and, in the universal gesture of self-blame, poked her finger at her temple, cocked her thumb and flicked the finger to mean the blast. Then she linked her arm in mine and gently drew me back to the table.

———

And yet, of course, comfort is real, and comes from other people. Foremost is a husband who was there for me every moment, rock-solid willing to be my wailing wall, who never expected or exacted any payment for it whatsoever; who understood how suddenly our lives changed course, and how long it takes to redirect the heart.

The effort of friends, acquaintances, and strangers, too—however rote, however demanded by mere etiquette—reassembles the shattered survivor bit by bit. Eloquence is nice but not required. A postage stamp, an envelope, an e-mail, handwriting, a picture of a puppy or a rose—every ragtag scrap of sympathy and shared sorrow knits into a safety net of unimagined strength. Everyone says this, and anyone who hasn't experienced it suspects a whiff of sentimentality. Don't believe it. The classmate and the teacher who showed up at his memorial; the former girlfriend who shared her reminiscences; the Ranger who posted a tribute on the Web; the friend from his childhood who flew down from New York; the major who installed a plaque in Tim's honor in the Special Forces Museum; every evidence that his life touched the life of someone else is a piece of the puzzle that means going on.

From Cairo Tim's stepmother, Barbi, wrote about a camping trip with the boys when Tim was still "a skinny, bucktoothed theatre-kid." They pitched camp on a hilltop near an old Minnesota Indian camp. "The weather was ominous and the yellow sky got dark early...It was tornado season...We read Poe by lantern light under the windwhipped, dripping canvas. Two terrified, small white faces and Walter with his scotch. The night wasn't too scary for Tim. He took the experience and made it a lifestyle."

Style was what Tim always admired in Barbi, and the pride was mutual. He had, she said, "imagination and flair, compassion and integrity; and I envied him for it. Adventure has lost some luster this week. I will miss him."

———

As soon as we were back from Namibia, John McBride called, wondering whether we wanted a memorial service in Tallahassee, offering to take the burden of preparation off our hands. I said no; I was too exhausted to go through it again. But within a few days I realized this was badly wrong. This too was Tim's home. He had lived here a dozen years, and off and on for thirty. He had prowled this little woods and helped build a tree house in it, long since fallen. He had taught Peter's daughter Anne to scuba dive in this pool and sat on its verge reading hour after hour in the sun. We needed to say goodbye *here* on this ground. The ground needed to say goodbye.

We put a notice in the *Tallahassee Democrat* and once again chose music from Haydn to Leonard Cohen, set up tables. I framed and set out thirty pictures of Tim from the day of his birth to the January snapshot, this last having by now been published in at least five newspapers in three countries. When I thought of how this would have displeased him I was angry: *then don't die.*

Elizabeth Dewberry filled the pool with floating candles, McBride and his father Blan spoke eloquently of Tim's life, Bob Butler read passages about him from my early essays, I read again the Jarrell poem, substituting for "I love you" Tim's deep-voice throwaway, "Love y', Mom!" Seventy or so sat on plastic chairs on the deck, or stood at the railing—Tim's dentist of thirty years backed into a candle and set his jacket tail on fire—and from the boom box in the balmy dark Alex's voice belted over the viburnum and the scuppernong vine:

> *Don't feel happy and I don't feel sad, no,*
> *Just lost the best friend I'll ever have.*
> *He was my brother, and I loved him so,*
> *Times long gone, pain lingers on and on,*
> *And I know…*
>
> *I wanna go home, wanna go home,*
> *Wanna go ho-o-o-me where I belong…*

Any direct address of the reality—condolence, conversation, rite—cocooned me in remoteness, and it would not be wrong to say I took joy in this evening. I accepted and arranged the food and flowers, hugged and chatted with Tim's friends and mine, and laughed with the colleague who said, meaning to praise my strength, "Janet throws a good party." I remember it with gratitude.

But in that same spot, later, the plastic Kmart *chaise longue* on the lip of the pool undid me. So often Tim lay on it inconsequentially bronzing, reading heroic trash. I liked the sight of him there because he was handsome, and because when he was a boy I could not afford a pool, so it was good to know that when he came home he had pleasure of it. At no time soever did I consider that sight precious. That he read adventure novels exasperated me. I was sometimes impatient for him to vacate my *chaise*.

Now I rose and plunged into the cold, cleaved it with fingers forked, driving myself through the wet, seeing him swim the earth.

5.

"You'll never understand," Stuart says, whose son hanged himself in a Florida hospital. "You have to stop yourself going down that road." But a therapist friend, says, "You need to come to some understanding that is satisfying to *you.*" And this seems the truer of the two.

Peter's daughter Anne, eighteen, comes to spend a couple of days with us, asking, "Why did he do it?" A stocky, mouse-haired, and gregarious child, she has transformed herself into a willowy blond beauty, wary, aloof. We struggle in conversation with her. We worry about anorexia. But she loved Tim, and now is baffled. "Why?" My answer, "He was disillusioned with the war," seems paltry, almost a refusal to answer. We are all disillusioned with the war.

I walk along a deserted beach at dawn under a dull sky, shouting at the surf: *you thought you were such a hero, you think it's so tough to pull a trigger, didn't I tell you, all the courage is in keeping on!?* Then anger topples into its opposite, into awe-full mourning not at my loss of Tim but at Tim's loss of the world: *you loved this; everything to do with it, boats and scuba and sun and surf and sand. Don't you remember how you loved it? How could you give it up?*

———

This pattern recurs. Again, another-gain. Peter and I clean the attic, tossing boxes of paperbacks, mildewed tents, khaki socks, camouflage shirts. I fume that there's so much military

48

gear—rifles, handguns, canteens, parachute jackets, matches in clever waterproof cases, several hundred pounds of ammunition. In my attic! Yet on Mother's Day I come across a freshman essay written at the University of Michigan, describing how coming home for Christmas really was coming home for him; how his mother went slightly bonkers over the holidays; how all his life she let him choose how to be himself and so had become his friend—"something not all kids can claim." I sit clutching these two pages of ruled notepaper among the detritus of a life.

Peter and I stand on a concrete slab in hundred-degree sun while workmen with a giant forklift retrieve three crates from a storage warehouse, pry them open, and spread out the contradictory stuff of a post-boomer bachelor pad. The suits are finely tailored, but the furniture tends to bricks 'n' boards. There's a high-tech coffee pot and a battered bunch of pans, an expensive-looking contraption for making bullets and a castoff couch. More guns, more ammo, and a delicate routing tool. It's so little to represent a life. So much of it is junk. I remember that it seemed my father, too, left paltry evidence of his rich existence.

We choose a few clothes that might fit Tim's friends, the antique maps and ebony and malachite carvings to fulfill his bequests. We entrust the guns to an Army friend. Among the boxes I find a folder of Army forms delivering up assessments of his work: "singularly outstanding...initiative, knowledge, and sound judgment...can excel at a myriad of simultaneous tasks...his commander's strong right arm...best Reserve officer I have seen come into this headquarters...a true professional...vital and key element on several pending real-world operational deployments...absolutely outstanding...top 5 percent of all officers I have ever known...should be assigned to command a Special Forces Operational Detachment Alpha." These are things he would never have shown me, parts of his life I would have gone to my grave not seeing except that I am sitting here surrounded by stacks of boxes, left to disperse his "effects."

———

Memorial Day weekend Peter buys me a sheet of gold cardboard and I make a pentagonal star and tape it in the window. Remembering that symbol from my early childhood in Phoenix during World War II, I feel a bitter reach to all those mothers who "willingly sacrificed," which I do not.

I dream there are little white grubs in my hair. I pick one out and try to crush it with my fingernail, but it gives plumply and recovers. In the dream I am holding a heavy computer battery, and these grubs also spill out of one end. It is urgent that I kill them, so I spray and dab the copper filaments with poison, then enclose it in a plastic bag. I carry this to an upstairs balcony and, my bare feet planted on red tile, look out through a Spanish arch at children playing in a courtyard below. Their play is dangerous. I want to warn them but feel I can't be heard or understood.

I cancel subscriptions and return the offers of credit, the alumni news, that still come to our house because this was Tim's only American address. Each time I write "cancel" or "deceased" I feel complicit in the erasure of my son. I do his posthumous taxes raging, because it isn't *right* that a parent should have to do this; it should be the other way around! I send with the tax forms an embossed certificate: *Cause of death: Gunshot: Head injury, skull fracture, brain laceration.* The words pulse on the page.

From Tim's gear I salvage a road sign stolen as a teenage

prank. Now when I look up from my desk I see pictures of Peter with toddler Anne walking among the dunes, of Alex post-punk in a blue shirt in front of a striped canopy, of Tim as he sat at the kitchen table on the last day I saw him alive: smiling, bearded, blue-eyed, beautiful. Beside them, clipped and laminated from the *New York Times*, an Iraqi father prostrate over the coffin of his son. Above these the pilfered sign: CAUTION: THE WEARING OF HARD HATS IS REQUIRED ON THIS JOB.

————

Tim left an informal will bequeathing everything to Birgitt aside from an appended list of people who were to choose a memento. He had a pistol and rifle collection and a modest store of maps, paintings, and African carvings. It was poignant and telling how this list divided and how, therefore, Tim saw us: his children, his half-brother Ben and his Army friend Rob were to choose guns; his stepmother, brother, half-sister, John McBride, and I were to receive artworks. The "everything" left to Birgitt included the mortgaged house and no more than enough money in their joint account to finance a frugal year. According to RONCO his life was not insured.

Some time in early June, Birgitt told me that she had been seeing a psychiatrist in Windhoek, a Dr. Reinhardt Sieberhagen, who volunteered that Tim's behavior in the last few weeks of his life exhibited the classic symptoms of post-traumatic stress disorder. The obsession with the news from Iraq and the safety of his men, the guilt toward them, the irritability, the sleeplessness, the drinking, the arousal, the hyper-vigilance toward Neal, the shaking on the ladder, the contradictory projection of his plans—all pointed to PTSD. Sieberhagen was willing to testify to a posthumous diagnosis, though he must clearly acknowledge that he had not seen Tim himself.

We agreed that I should go speak to the Veterans' Administration, which turned out to be housed in a defunct but charmingly refurbished Tallahassee railway station. The major, who gave me a leisurely hour, had an air both tough and grandfatherly, a burly, sympathetic Old Soldier who had seen it all. He loaded my arms with forms. He told me that in order for Tim's widow and children to get VA benefits, we would have to show not simply that Tim had PTSD, but that the relevant trauma had occurred while he was active and deployed. He picked my brain about Tim's experience in the Army. In Bosnia, Congo, Angola. Maiming? Bombing? Death seen up close? He said that the road to VA benefits was tortuous, that most people wearied of it long before they were assessed, and that lawyers in the endless process of reviews and appeals called it "the hamster wheel."

Tim's professional reticence was a hindrance now. He had spoken to Birgitt in cryptic, nearly encrypted, terms about a plane that had crashed or disappeared off the coast of Congo. A Tallahassee friend thought he had been in that crash, and that the soldier beside him had died in it. Birgitt was of the impression he had been assigned to investigate. Could that be the "real-world deployment" mentioned in his assessments? But if his cageyness indicated some official secret, she wasn't likely to learn about it from an official source.

I searched through his early letters looking for evidence of trauma. What I found instead was a kind of grim self-satisfaction when things were tough. From Ranger training he boasted that a dry rations pack "seems like a six-course meal" and that the Ranger Instructor had told them that their bodies would go quickly into starvation mode and they would start burning muscle.

> ...*It was a smoker!...I got about 3 hours sleep in four days. Moving through the night...I'm exhausted but it really doesn't seem to matter...The next 2 weeks will be in the swamps and rivers...All we think about is food!...There were lots of mushrooms in the mountains and I kept thinking about sautéed mushrooms in butter...Love, your short-haired somewhat skinnier son..."*

From Schofield Barracks in Hawaii he wrote that he felt his body had been "put through a pipe-threader," that his four rucksacks felt as if they were cutting through his shoulder, and that his LBE (whatever that was) had "rubbed [his] ass raw." His tone ranged from jaunty irony ("As they say here, the beauty of the place is inversely proportional to the weight of the rucksack and the distance traveled") to defiant pride ("An infantry officer earns every salute and privilege he gets.") to griping ("I've been tasked with playing in a Command Post Exercise...next week I'll be up all night doing dumb stuff so that the general's staff learns something.")

Tim wanted to be tested and wanted to test himself. He told me more than once that he wanted to be the "go-to guy." What he liked was "to be given a problem no one else could solve, and then solve it." In fact the only time I could remember any hardship that was not expressed as half-proud grousing involved not trauma but the long and debilitating hassle that led to his leaving the Army.

After ROTC at University of Florida, Tim was commissioned as a lieutenant and joined the regular Army at Fort

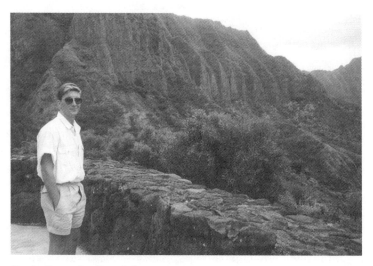

On the Banzai Pipeline, Oahu, 1990

Benning, attended Ranger and Paratrooper training from there, and was given the lucky assignment of Hawaii.

In the spring of 1991 I visited him on the island of Oahu. I found him fit and blithe. He was squandering his pay on a sleek black Nissan SRX in which he drove me through the mountains. He rented with two or three other young Army bachelors a spacious if shabby two-story house perched over the Banzai Pipeline. While they were at work I pursued tourist pleasures in a rental car, or cooked and scoured for them to hoots of appreciation and derision—"We don't know how to make coffee in a clean pot!" Like Tim they affected a *yes-ma'am* politesse; like him they were gung ho for Operation Desert Storm, which they saw as the necessary defense of a victimized Kuwait. When I said I believed war didn't work, and that this one was being fought to protect oil rather than Arabs, they expressed their incredulity in friendly terms. Tim smiled indulgently. It was all quite jolly.

But over the next year I began to hear the wear in Tim's voice. When I called and asked how he was, he would say, "Survivin', survivin'." This too was an Army tic, but it was too often succeeded by a litany of stress. The lieutenant colonel who was commanding officer of his battalion had appointed him executive officer (later battalion adjutant), which meant administration, personnel, management, and logistics. The CO said, "Eysselinck, I know you want to be in the field. But I've got to have somebody in the office who can *write*." Tim had reported this conversation expecting me to laugh, and I had. He'd waited for me to say, "Your genes will out." And I had.

But he suffered from not being in the field. Indoors grated on him, the computer tasks he performed with such facility dragged him down. Worse, the colonel seemed increasingly incapable of making a decision. While his comrades were humping a hundred pounds over the lava fields, Tim was stuck arranging some ceremonial dinner, and the CO would wake him in the middle of the night having changed the venue, or the menu, or the invitation list. No sooner had Tim put through the orders for equipment, or commendation, or war game teams, than the CO would change his mind and then change it back again. When the orders came through for the company to be deployed to Iraq, the colonel seemed to rev up to wheel-spinning neurosis. Now Tim had no sleep not because he was digging trenches but because he was called out and hauled out to rescind last Tuesday's work. On the phone he alternated between rage and listlessness. He had gone to the chaplain for counseling. He thought the colonel was a danger to the troops. He thought the level of indecision would endanger all their lives on the battlefield. "Mom, I've been a warrior without a war the whole time here. But if I go to Iraq as his EO I think I'll be psych-med-evac'ed out within six months."

This clash resulted in a less than stellar annual report from the CO—by which I don't mean bad; I mean less than stellar, upper-mediocre. Tim was not used to such assessments and couldn't stand it. He thought he should appeal. He thought he should report his CO's dangerous irresolution. But that would mean going over the colonel's head, an iffy move in a rigid hierarchy. The chaplain whose advice he sought agreed both that it was the right thing to do and that it was risky. The alternative was to resign.

He resigned, finally, because, he said, he felt he was going crazy. At no time was this, nor did I suspect it was, cold feet about the war. On the contrary, he said the hardest thing he ever did was to put his men on the plane and watch them fly off to Desert Storm without him. It was I who, worried about his emotional state, was nevertheless grateful he had distanced himself from the Army.

The executive officer who replaced Tim under that CO was psych-med-evac'ed out of Iraq within six months.

———

Tim came home to Tallahassee, shared a house with John McBride, and went to work as a trainee broker for Dean Witter. He had met, on vacation at home, a young woman I'll call Jewel. Born of a Punjabi Sikh family but raised in Tallahassee, Jewel was tall, dark, and stunningly beautiful. Jewel and Tim had known each other a little in high school. Now they seemed quickly serious. She and I lunched. I went to dinner with her family. Anne, who had a crush on Tim, transferred it to Jewel. Peter and I began to imagine a blue-eyed black-haired grandchild.

But the job was everything Tim most despised. He would

show up at his lunch hour, impeccably suited, fuming at the pointless cant of his corporate education. "Those sleazebags. Half of it is common sense and the other half is a con." In the attic after he died I found a personality test he had taken for the job. Its analysis was consonant with those lunchtime rants. The assessment found him "highly motivated" in spite of "some (possibly unexpressed) nagging doubts about the validity of a sales career," observed that when it came to peddling "financial products" to friends and family he "may find sales prospecting ethically troublesome and/or professionally unacceptable."

In retrospect, the smarmy jargon justifies his disgust. But at the time, I worried about him, and I also got impatient with him. His anger seemed over the top. He seemed to be roiling to no purpose. I don't know if it occurred to me then that coming from that CO to this enterprise was out-of-the-flypaper into-the-taffy-trap. It was several months before he was offered a job in security for the multinationals in Cameroon. And although Jewel would not pull up stakes, quit her job, and go with him, he was outta here for the first of several times to Africa.

———

I could plot a pattern in the way Tim's energy and purpose waxed and waned. He told me several times, perhaps half a dozen, warningly, that he was willing to die for his country if he was called upon. He even self-consciously boasted he could see himself heading heroically into battle. The times I saw him most unhappy he was wearing a suit and tie—as a Dean Witter trainee, and later as headhunter for a computer firm. I think it was the latter time—late nineties—that he said one afternoon out of the blue, "If it wasn't for what it'd do to you, I'd kill myself." I was shocked but—is it accurate to say *inattentive*? Perhaps there was a fundamental parental sense in which I wanted to deny his anguish, could not take it on. Above all, knowing I had myself been deeply down and yet won through to a happy life, I assumed he would do the same after the *sturm* of youth had passed.

And now I remembered that thirty years ago I wrote a story called "Extra Days," imagined, as such stories often are, out of several autobiographical scraps. It was about the single mother of a ten-year-old boy who is jealous of her live-in lover. The boy threatens to kill himself with "pungee sticks" like those he's heard about in Vietnam. The boy saves a crab from the beach but later accidentally kills it. And flings himself on the mother's boyfriend for solace—

> *"... because Garth was the fixer, the doer, the one for whom the sea was alive. She, herself, was not at all reassured; not reconciled. She was only, standing at a little distance from their private enterprise, flooded with unabashed pity for her son, because he was her son and her sort, for whom the longest thing to learn and the hardest to remember, for whom the decision of every day, never finally made nor wholly understood, would be how willing he was, after all, to live."*

This story was written in my recovery from post-divorce depression. It moves me with memory of that time, and of how, then, I had identified with his pain. But that he was "my sort" verged on presumption, since in the end he had not been, after all, so willing.

6.

Three or four times a week I turned right on Meridian and right again on Bradford to reach Thomasville Road. This meant that I passed Bradford Court just under the second-story entrance of the last apartment Tim occupied in America: the driveway climbing behind a hedge, a camphor tree, gray-washed cedar siding, an outside staircase with a tropical plant—someone else's now. It was a desensitization course. At first the sight took me by surprise and I exhibited all the signs of fight-or-flight: heartbeat, sweat glands, stomach, breathing pattern, hackles. Then I learned to prepare myself as I made the turn, and could control my breathing, leave the steering wheel dry beneath my palms. By mid-June when we left for London I could negotiate Bradford without a hitch.

Why did it not occur to me that I would have to negotiate England too?

————

It's unfashionable now to be an Anglophile—so sixties, so literary canon, so toff and twee. Much better to be in love with Krakow or admire the Thais.

But I'm stuck with it. My Anglophilia began in southern California at the age of seven or eight with the sight of "Pinkie" and "Blue Boy" at the Huntington Art Gallery. These were the first "high art" I had seen in a childhood dominated by *Looney Tunes*, and I like to believe that as a child I was as

awed by the artistry as the romanticism. Later I gravitated—
who knows why?—more to George Eliot than Emily Dick-
inson, more to Joseph Conrad than Herman Melville. I went
to England first in 1958 as a Marshall scholar to Cambridge
University and later, during my first marriage, spent six years
in a Sussex village called Westmeston so small that it didn't
even have a pub. Florida State had a London program too,
and the boys and I had come back to England more than
once for that. When my father died in 1986 he left me twenty
thousand dollars that I used as down payment on a one-room
London flat. Peter and I (we married in 1993) moved up in
1998 to another, small by American standards but big enough
that we both could write there, and by now it was our habit to
come every summer. Alex had returned to England when he
was sixteen (the only one of the family to hold a British pass-
port, he never did become American) and was partnered with
Tricia Howard from Hertfordshire. Their very English daughters were, at the time of Tim's death, Eleanor Janet, eight years
old, and Holly Catherine, six.

It was solace to see them, and I believed that England
itself would distract me. Tim had only been there once as an
adult, when he was stationed in Germany and his niece Eleanor was born. He was not *present* in London, or so I unthink-
ingly believed, so I would not be reminded of him.

Why didn't I foresee that his childhood would come
flooding back?

There are ways upon ways to keep realization from seep-
ing in. I was still learning that the appropriate emotion is
not on tap, that it always comes in a rush just when I think
either that I'm handling everything or else that I'm a callous
fraud. A friend visited us in London and I showed him the
essays and pictures of Tim's life that had appeared in the *St.*

Petersburg Times. He wept while I sat unmoved, or moved to cut a piece of pie. I thought: *three months and I'm over it. I must be an unnatural mother.* Some hours later I sat on the Underground across from a young man who looked nothing at all like Tim—a bluff, black-haired sort—but who had intense, alive blue eyes. My lungs imploded. I could not draw breath. Lines came to me that I had learned at half Tim's age and hadn't thought of for thirty years:

> *... That you were gone, not to return again—*
> *Read from the back page of a paper, say,*
> *Held by a neighbor on a subway train...*

And those were followed by a surge of the girlish reverence, long since repudiated, that I had felt for Edna St. Vincent Millay:

> *... And entering with relief some quiet place*
> *Where never fell his foot or shone his face*
> *I say, 'There is no memory of him here!'*
> *And so stand stricken, so remembering him.*

The images of Tim's Sussex childhood lay in wait in the accents, in the flintstones, in teapots and Wellington boots and Matchbox toys. I would see a double-decker bus on any ordinary London day, and Tim would appear in the living room of the Sussex house, on the shoulders of my agent's son, also named Tim, shouting "Double-decker Timothy! Double-decker Timothy!"

The memories came in random order and like all memories of him were corrupted with the awareness of his death. Peter asked, "When were you first aware of his reticence?" And

I could feel—my arms could remember it—Tim squirming, arching, seven months old and wanting to get *away*, whereas Alex was still asking for a cuddle at five or six years.

It was when he was about seven months that Walter and I left Tim in Ghent with "Grandma Belgium" and took a week's vacation to Ireland. On the way we visited David Daiches, who had been my supervisor at Cambridge and was now the Professor of English and American Studies at the new "glass brick" University of Sussex. We learned that the University was looking for a director of a proposed Arts Centre, and Daiches said that if Walter could obtain the post, he would put me up for a lectureship in English. It was a heady time—Walter was also offered directorship of the Flemish-language National Theatre of Belgium—and after a few months it was arranged. We moved to Sussex in the summer of 1965, rented a bungalow in a tract, started searching for a permanent home, and began our jobs. There was one angst-ridden false start at finding someone to look after Tim, and then we encountered and hired a lovely soft-natured young woman, married and later herself pregnant, who would bus to the top of the road where I'd pick her up every morning, go in to teach my classes, and then take her back to the bus stop mid-afternoon.

In that first year Walter began work with the architects for the Gardner Centre. He organized concerts and exhibitions. He directed the first of many plays. I studied hard to keep up with eight or nine tutorials a week. I set up a costume shop for the theatre. I finished my third novel. We entertained prospective "Friends of the Gardner Centre." I got pregnant. Walter wrapped the car around a telephone pole and spent three weeks in plastic surgery (the shape of his jaw permanently squared). Through all which Tim seemed to thrive.

That year we searched for a house, and after months of indecision, surges of enthusiasm, and cold feet, we bought for more than we could afford a bleak brick box on two acres of rolling land under the South Downs. The house had big cube rooms smudged ochre with twenty years of ash, and many mullioned windowpanes of which one hundred eight were broken. But these windows looked onto a garden that had been tended for thirty years by a Mr. Ashley who had designed it so that no prospect would ever be free of flowers, and it would yield food in every month. A stand of bamboo and flowering cherry, lawns reaching to the ruin of a tennis court, lush rose beds and an orchard, and two thirds of an acre *laid to* (as I learned to say) vegetables and fruit. You could see from this garden no other house, only fields cropped short by sheep and cows, sloping gently away or, beyond the road, rising to the crest of the Downs.

The house had been built in the thirties for the farm bailiff of the local manor, had been requisitioned for troops during the Second World War, was thereafter turned into a maternity hospital, and had for twenty years been inhabited by a minor noblewoman of the county and a servant of Dickensian intrigue. This servant had finally inherited the house, but in such condition that only we wanted it. No system or surface was livable. The floor had to be jacked up, the wiring replaced, the coal furnace pulled out, the cupboards scrubbed of webs and grime. I was seven months pregnant when we moved in. I painted walls while Walter did the ceilings—of a hall eighteen feet square, a living room twenty by thirty, a "staff flat" that we would rent out to pay for Mr. Ashley's gardening time. The Daicheses lent us two thousand pounds for the essential work, but we lived with broken windows, splintered floors, and a single electrical socket. The heating system was installed in cold November a couple of days before Tobyn Alexander was born in the smallest of the seven bedrooms.

Over the next five years the house was gradually transformed into livable space while the marriage fell into disrepair. Walter had, on the surface, complementary ambitions in theatre and writing, and politics in sync with mine. He liked Americans, and I was sentimental about all things Continental. My friend Julia once observed that we'd have been fine if we hadn't thought we had to be in love—because temperamentally we were at odds. Walter needed directorial power not only in the theatre but at home. His career was all-consuming. Our best times together centered in some way around his professional success. It was very early days of women's lib, which at first held little attraction for me. I genuinely loved the domestic, and I thought I could handle the writing, teaching, and mothering. But we quarreled about time and money, about who was to cook, whom we should entertain, whether I should have my own car, whether I needed his permission to buy clothes for the boys, whether I was to visit my mother in Arizona. We drank too much. The quarrels became bitter and on occasion physical. I fell into an ugly pleasure when I could predict his autocratic stance.

Nevertheless, most of my images of Tim in those years are of the garden, of his intently helping Mr. Ashley wind the strings for the green beans or poke the holes to plant potato eyes. He would run to meet Mr. Ashley at the top of the drive in the morning and ride the handlebars down to the garden shed. Mr. Ashley was infinitely patient. Tim was happy too with the series of graduate students who rented the flat, with Brian who came on weekends to replace those broken windows, and with Tricia, a plump, sunny-natured country girl who became my friend as well.

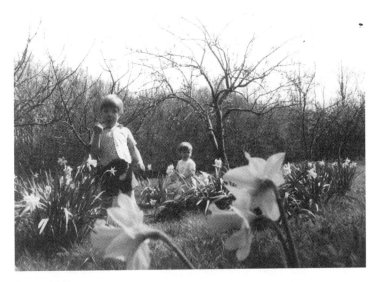

Sussex, 1968

So what now seems portentous must be placed (this is also what Birgitt said of Tim's last days) against a background of normal energy and cheer, precisely the qualities I strove with increasing difficulty to present to the boys.

I have a black-and-white snapshot of Tim and his little brother, both of them tow-headed and long-lashed, standing in an orchard full of daffodils. I also own a color photograph taken in the African savanna, of my grown elder son kneeling beside the carcass of an antelope, accompanied by his wiry Cameroonian guides. One image I hold in my head is of Tim, White Hunter, being mocked by these guides because, rigorous about the rules of the sport, he was unwilling to poach on government land. They thought he was afraid. Now, looking at the toddler in the daffodils, I can see the clear lineaments of the hunter's face. But squatting beside him I had no premonition of which planes, tilts, colors of that cherub

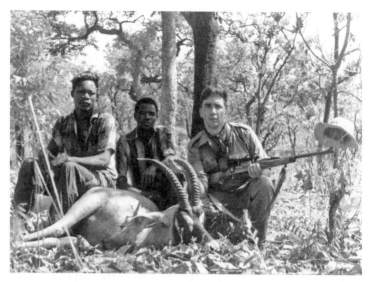

Cameroon, Africa c. 1993

head would survive. Looking back, I can see clearly that his passion for little plastic planes and tanks, the bags of khaki-colored soldiers on whose webbing belts he layered a patina with a one-hair brush, the catalogues of insignias of rank—in all that, I can see that his direction was early set. But I was a first-time parent. I thought all boys played soldier. Toby-Alex liked model planes too, and it did not absolutely register that by the time he was ten he had given up soldier stuff and gone into other fantasies, to Dungeons and Dragons and from thence to the Society for Creative Anachronism, whereas Tim never altered an iota from the interests that burgeoned in that ramshackle house.

The university was fifteen minutes by car over the Ditchling Beacon with its heart-lifting lookout point on the top of the downs. But we had only one car and some difficulty making our schedules jibe. At four Tim started at the university pre-school, so the three of us would drive in mornings and then carpool the return trip, alternating with the parents of Gavin Paine, who lived in Ditchling village. One winter day Tim, Gavin, and I were to be driven home by Walter's secretary, when a deep and sudden blizzard covered Sussex. Greba's car would not mount the hill. She turned to take us the long way 'round but the car coughed and hiccupped to a standstill on the frozen highway, and we had to hitch a ride into Lewes station hoping to get a bus.

England, which can handle war with pluck and verve, is notoriously undone by snow. Neither trains nor buses were running. Nobody was going anywhere. You could see on people's faces the pleasant surprise that, after all, nothing they had to do mattered very much. Strangers bought each other biscuits and cups of tea. Neither Gavin nor Tim had gloves, and I proposed we should climb the sidewalk into Lewes to buy them some. I can see them, marching stiff-armed up the hill in the deep snow, *left-right, left-right,* Tim counting out the orders, Russian soldiers in the Eastern Campaign. Was he really so aware of World War II, at the age of barely five? It seems unlikely, and yet by then he knew, which I do not now, the difference between the Fokker, Hurricane, and Hunter fighter planes. And the memory is quite specific: Russian soldiers on Germany's Eastern Front.

That day it took us eight hours to go eight miles. In early evening a bus made it as far as Plumpton Green, where the local pub owner was brewing hot chocolate and hot toddies for the stranded. Tim balked at the threshold. "My daddy says children are not allowed in pubs. It's the *law*." We convinced him, with difficulty, that an emergency overwrote the rules.

Tim's relationship to his father was devoted and full of longing in these years. Walter, working out of a quonset hut, trying to attract artists to a "Centre" that had as yet no center, was overtired and under pressure. He was in any case an anxiously ambitious man, for whom a career in the English-speaking theatre was the golden fleece. In the first few years of Tim's life he had enjoyed the role of father. Now he was increasingly preoccupied. I think Alex had the easier time of it because from the beginning he had few expectations of his father, whereas Tim depended on attention that was not forthcoming.

We were house-poor, too, and living in several ways beyond our means. There were weekends when we sent visitors away with armloads of squash and fennel but could not afford to stand a round of drinks at the local pub. Sometimes when we came home at midnight from the Gardner Centre, weary with imminent production, Mr. Ashley would have left word that the peas were ready; and I would go into the garden with a flashlight to pick them, would stay up all night canning or freezing. How could I let them go to waste? When the production was over, I would cook for cast parties, thick soups and mountains of sliced vegetables and berry parfaits. How could I not share such wealth? I washed rivers of mud down the sink until the septic tank backed up.

Out of Tim's passion for trucks and trains I wrote a children's book, and we made friends with the illustrator, John Vernon Lord, and his wife and daughters, who also lived in Ditchling. One spring afternoon Tim and Toby and I sat in their garden having tea in the sun. The girls showed Tim their bicycle and within ten minutes he could ride it, balancing down the paths through the hedgerows over the hummocky ground. Home again, I told Walter that Tim was ready for a bike. Walter said we couldn't afford it. I countered that a bike cost less than a case of wine—this was a familiar pattern of argument. But this one, which ended in Walter's decreeing that I could look in the second-hand stores, took on symbolic weight for me. I let the anger fester. I bought the used bicycle, but the chain slipped and could not be repaired. Mr. Ashley would try to fix it. Tim would ride for ten feet or so, get off, get out his wrench, tighten the bolt again. Ride, slip, wrench. He would sit frustrated on the path in the dirt, heels of his hands in his eyes, trying not to cry. And, watching from the kitchen window, I would seethe.

And yet. Once when Walter was in Belgium directing a television play, I wrote my parents that toddler Tim had wandered the house looking behind doors, sadly chanting, "Papa all gone." Two years later when Walter was away, Tim wet the bed three or four nights in a row. I reassured him it was a common thing, but on the way to the station to pick Walter up, he said, "You see, when my daddy's not here, well, I don't feel so sure about things. I don't feel so sure about the *world*." Insecurity never had a clearer articulation. I determined at that moment that I could not take this boy away from his father.

And yet. After two or three exciting Christmases in the Sussex house, when socks and sauce pans were turned into surprises, when Walter made gift wrapping into a fine art; there were holidays when he came home so drunk that he couldn't get up for Christmas morning. Eh-las-bas!—a handsome retard of an Irish setter named after a favorite jazz lyric—could not be dissuaded from chasing sheep in the neighboring field. When he had been out thus sinning, Walter would take him into the front cloak room to "kick some sense into him." There was no shielding the boys from those howls. (When I arrived home in Arizona, after elaborate machinations to keep the truth from my ailing mother, she greeted me at the door with "You've left him, haven't you? I knew it when he kicked the dog.")

It must have been New Year's Day 1970, Walter in Belgium again directing, that Tim was playing with his paratrooper Action Man. The man-doll was a foot tall in those days, with a plethora of armored-car equipment that we were gradually acquiring. The paratrooper was a working model in the sense that, dropped from a height, it would waft to ground under the buoyancy of the 'chute. The balcony around the big hall was just right. Tim would drop the figure and then race down the stairs trying to beat it down.

I was used to standing white-knuckled at the kitchen sink while the boys climbed sixty feet into the horse chestnut in the orchard—chanting to myself, "Boys have to climb trees, boys have to climb trees"—so the parachuting game didn't seem especially dangerous. Toby was apt to wander into the field among the cows or up to the snowy highway (once he walked on the window-glass skylight, once he narrowly escaped a plunging roof tile), but Tim was on the whole thoughtful and sane, and it didn't register with me that he was in his stockinged feet. On the tenth or dozenth jump, Tim raced as usual down the stairs, lost his footing on the second to the bottom step, and fell back, hitting his head on the tread.

I held him while he cried, but the crying went on and on, so I called the doctor, who said if he still seemed upset or disoriented after half and hour, to take him into the Children's Hospital in Brighton. I built a fire in the hall and sat with him and Toby on a blanket in front of it. After half an hour Tim still seemed weepy and "wonky," some of his movements random. We had a young couple living in the flat, and the woman took charge of Toby while the man drove me into town—luckily, because I could not have handled Tim while driving. He thrashed and pulled against my arms, screaming obscenities I didn't know he knew.

At the hospital the nurses described his state as "irritable," while he flailed against the sidebars of the bed, pissing yellow puddles of rage. Once the doctor arrived, Tim shouted, "You turn on the lights! I told you turn on the lights!" and both of us realized he was blind. This blindness and "irritability" lasted for fifteen hours, and I was asked to sign a release for brain surgery before I left by taxi to get back to Toby.

Next morning when we arrived Tim was sitting up in bed eating corn flakes and watching "The Magic Roundabout," annoyed I had left him in this stupid place. For the next week I was charged with "keeping him quiet," which I (barely) managed, in a wry demonstration that I am better in a crisis than a slog.

Did I fail? Was there some invisible damage to his brain that would show up in adulthood, the way my broken tailbone surfaced as lumbar pain? No. Silly and pretentious. Still. Boxers and football players decades later suffer the results of trauma. Discussing the head wounds of Iraq veterans, Dr. Greg O'Shannon of the Brain Injury Association says that concussion can jar the frontal lobe in such a way as to produce "chronic disease, just like diabetes," and can effect depression, irritability, impulsivity.

———

Nineteen seventy-one was a year of crisis. The Gardner Centre, designed by Sean Kenny and Basil Spence, was built by now, a masterpiece of adaptability. It had housed successful concerts, exhibitions, and plays, but Walter's relations with the students and the actors were often rocky. For the summer production of 1971, he pulled off the coup of casting a famous television star in a two-hander, the other role to be played by Bernie Hopkins, with whom Walter had worked several times. Bernie was a brilliant actor and a bubbling favorite of us all, boys emphatically included. We had plenty of room in our sprawling house, and the actors' salaries were peanuts, so both the famous actor and Bernie were to stay with us through the rehearsal period.

A few weeks before rehearsals were to begin I had a phone call from a playwright friend, diffident, who said, well, it was none of his business, and he was sure I knew what I was doing, but did I realize that the Famous Star was a pederast with a penchant for young boys?

I said that I had heard this, but that I'd reasoned it this way: he would never be alone with them, Tim and Toby were *too* young, and in any case Famous, whatever his proclivities, had too much taste to betray his host.

All of these things were borne out, as was my naïveté. Famous was never alone with them, they were too young, he had too much taste; and yet for six weeks I stood by wringing my hands while this skillful actor in effect made love to them. He read them heroic tales of World War II; he built them a fort with a "suicide slide" (!) from the horse chestnut to the hawthorn hedge; he gave me instructions for the uniform bits I was to sew. It was all patently innocent boy-stuff, and when Tim or Toby said, "Isn't _____ wonderful, Mummy?" I had no option but to agree.

I did not know what to do. Walter's mind was always elsewhere. He was in negotiation with Michael Winner for a play, and Winner was out of Walter's league for power and its machinations. After morning rehearsal, Bernie and Famous would come back to the house while Walter spent long hours in the office and came home spewing his frustration, ignoring the boys as they ran to him. Famous continued to spin boy-magic, meanwhile requiring of me-his-hostess this kind of marmalade or that sort of citrus fruit that we could not afford. Bernie would shepherd the boys and me off to the Saturday market to distract us. Evenings when Famous and the boys were in bed and Walter was still at work, Bernie and I would sit in our robes gossiping, girls in a dorm. Of Famous, Bernie warned me, "There are gays who love men, and there are gays who hate women. Beware *la différence.*"

Six weeks in that situation is an arduous long time. Walter saw clearly what was going on, but, torn between outrage and ambition, like me he could point to no specific complaint. And then one morning saw him howling on the back step, "Get that man away from my children!" and Bernie and I both thought that murder was very literally possible.

Perhaps Bernie got Famous away—I don't remember how it happened that Walter and I were alone at the kitchen table, but I know that Walter said, "I can't stand sickness." I knew he was referring not to Famous but to the memory of his father's suicide, for which Walter still bitterly blamed him. I said, "Then don't *be* your father. Ask for help when you need it!" This was a lucky choice. He acquiesced. I called our GP, who drove out to the house, though by the time he arrived Walter had downed a half bottle of gin and was elegant, dismissive, full of slightly slurry charm. The doctor admitted him to hospital all the same, and knocked him out for thirty-six hours. Later he told me that he couldn't read Walter at all; he measured Walter's need by the level of stress he saw in me.

I felt in those days, and in the several succeeding months, that I was living with a dangerous machine I didn't know how to operate. It took me several months to see its effect on Tim. By fall he was in his third year at the Ditchling primary school, a four-room flintstone cottage arrived at through the local graveyard. Now two or three afternoons a week he would come home and hunch into me in tears. I would sit him on my lap and rock him for fifteen or twenty minutes while he sobbed. Up to this time I had thought him a rather serious but normal child, with the usual complement of temper, laughter, energy, and greed. Now he claimed that the kids at school all hated him. They always chose him last. They wouldn't play with him. His grief seemed all the more real because I was myself by then so unhappy.

I went to see his teacher, a tall, affable young man, who shook his head in surprise. "I haven't seen a sign of it. He seems perfectly popular to me." I asked him please to keep watch for a week; I'd be back. A week later I was back. The young man shook his head again. "It just isn't true, Mrs. Eysselinck. He's one of the popular ones. He plays normally, he's accepted. I mean—it just isn't *true*."

It may have been the next morning that I turned off the alarm, carried the paper up to Walter, dressed the boys, served Walter's egg, absorbed some complaint, snapped back at him, bundled the boys into the car, and drove to Hassocks to pick up the nanny—burning at the imbalance of labor—and realized that Tim was carried from breakfast every morning on this tide of anger. He deflected it onto the playground where he could both suffer it and bear it.

That afternoon as he sat on my lap, sobbing, I picked up a "Ladybird Book." Toby too climbed into my lap, and I read them the saccharine story about a British family's trip of discovery to the United States. It had the works—skyscrapers, cowboys, White House, Grand Canyon, Golden Gate—and ended with one of the children effusing, "It really *is* the land of the free and the home of the brave!" Specious. Mawkish. And all three of us now in tears.

Tim's school grief was not the tipping point of the marriage, which came some weeks later, requiring an escalation of marital melodrama and the fantasy of a romance on my part. But it effectively neutralized the notion of "staying for the children's sake."

7.

This is the nature of it. I fold a pair of Peter's socks off the drying rack in the London flat. I notice they have little gray clocks down the side. I go to him. "Are you okay with clocks in your socks? I thought you always wanted plain."

"Clocks in my socks? Clocks in my socks?" He laughs.

"Yes, this little woven pattern. It's known as a clock."

"I never heard of that."

"Yes, you did. You've forgotten. There was that mystery gift one year when Tim was home for Christmas—a rhinoceros clock. *Genuine quartz and brass rhinoceros clock,* something like that. I used a pair of socks as a clue for the clock and none of you got it."

"I remember. Tim won it. He always won."

"He *loved* the mystery gift."

"What happened to that clock? It wasn't in his stuff."

"How can you, how could he, love the mystery gift so much and kill himself?"

And I am washed over with angry grief.

———

That summer the plan had been for the British and Namibian cousins at last to meet. In Namibia I had insisted that Tim's family should come ahead, and now they arrived: Birgitt, Thyra, and Neal, bringing with them Neal's grandmother, Marienne, in place of Tim.

For ten days we scouted London with Alex, Tricia, Eleanor, and Holly. We saw *Stomp* and Princess Diana's Kensington playground and the Museum of Science; consumed quantities of lamb and gooseberry tart and ice lollies and best back rashers. Eleanor, eight, assumed the authority of a nanny over her toddler cousin. Neal figured out the Underground system and thrived on his unaccustomed freedom.

I was exhausted. I sat shoulders-sagging on the park bench while the children played. Having served up a dinner at noon, I would take to bed at two o'clock. Wandering the stalls at Camden Town market, my favorite Sunday outing, I found the weight of my handbag shot pain from my shoulder to my wrist and up the back of my head. I wanted only to get off my feet, out of my clothes, on the couch, in bed.

———

The three girls were as different from each other as Tim had been from Alex, but also impressed with the importance of their blood ties (curious how early this family awareness happens—*my cousin, my step-aunt, my great-uncle*) and also, no doubt, aware of their several places in the catastrophe.

Eleanor is dark-haired, appreciative, logical, and driven to excel. Holly at two years younger is blonde, sensitive, voluble, and given to fantasy. What the sisters had in common was an ability to amuse themselves and each other, to put greed and anger quickly aside, to go along with what was proposed—and these virtues were, recognizably, the result of a disciplined upbringing by Tricia and (amazing!) my punk-in-plain-clothes son.

But I worried about Thyra, who seemed pent with anger. I had little insight into what the children were going through. Grief, like depression, constricts the ability to empathize.

Thyra is one of the most beautiful children I have ever seen, so alarmingly smart that she has real, not recounted-to-her, memories of Peter and me when she was not quite a year old. But that summer she bit when angry, spat when thwarted, grasped and grabbed. She also disarmed passersby with chirping openness and turned a face of angelic innocence to one reprimand in three. Later, I was startled to find this description in a novel by Nadine Gordimer: "This bright and beguiling little girl is self-willed in excess of her size and approximate age, manipulative, a show-off in the spotlight of demanded attention and the next half hour gloweringly withdrawn." The character this passage describes is a black African adoptee, and we readers find her rather wonderful. But in London the summer after Tim's death I could not summon the energy for admiration.

One afternoon when Birgitt and I had gone to the corner shops, I was looking over vegetables in the grocer's outdoor bins while Birgitt, carrying Thyra, window-shopped the antique store next door. There was some altercation between mother and daughter, and just as the antique shop owner came outside, Thyra bit Birgitt on the shoulder, hard.

The woman reared back with a face of real (and also probably exaggerated) outrage. "What a *bad* girl!" she said. "You must never, *never* bite!"

"Don't worry, it didn't hurt," Birgitt trilled.

I went in and paid for my strawberries. Tim's childhood was in my head, and also his often-reiterated opinion that I'd been too permissive as a parent. "I appreciated the freedom, Mom," he would say, grinning but meaning it, "but my own kids will have more discipline." I counted out my change. My permissiveness, I thought, would never have run to allowing a child to bite.

Later at home, recounting it in laughter, Birgitt said, "Thyra absolutely charmed the woman!" And no doubt in the end she had.

I can't remember whether it was that evening or another that Alex and Birgitt debated discipline. Birgitt contended that the English stunted and repressed their children, and that the reason was ultimately that the island is so small. Children, like plants, she said, "must have room to grow and spread their branches." Alex countered that plants need pruning to reach their potential of growth and health. That was the gist of the argument, which, however, lasted through a couple of bottles of wine, during which the garden metaphor composted and turned rank. Birgitt said, "You sound just like your brother. I can't tell you how many arguments we had about this!"

It was a full year before I realized that Thyra's tenacity and her tantrums did not represent her personality, and that her behavior was skewed and strained by her father's death. A year later, Peter and I spent a delightful weekend with her, in and out of the pool and hot tub—"Opa Peter! Look at me!"—life popping from her like popcorn, pop! pop! pop! She sobbed at our parting, buckets, howls. "I'll never see you again!" Then I recognized that in the normal course of things, a child experiences a friend or parent going away and coming back again, going and coming, and learns to trust in the return. But in the third year of Thyra's short life her father had left for Iraq, returned, left, returned, and then left forever. The rebuilding of her trust would take many partings, years of returns.

———

After Tim's family had gone back to Namibia we settled into a quieter routine. I had bad days—clumsy, effortful, itchy with inauthenticity—and then for no apparent reason, equilibrium. One afternoon we stripped the dining room table, gently, with steel wool, but nevertheless at some point penetrated the surface of the veneer. I found myself trivially wanting to claw back time to make it whole again. And I realized that this was not the case with Tim. The fact of his death loomed so solid that there was no sense of wishing to go back. There was no *back*. And yet, and yet—this very acknowledgement set up the familiar round of regret: if I had called and reached him that afternoon, wouldn't I have heard the trouble in his voice? Could I have made a difference?

Often, in the past few years, I had said, "We're so lucky. I know it can all change..." But what I anticipated was old age, predictable afflictions: that Peter might have a stroke, that I might get cancer or my heart might fail. I remembered how Aunt Jessie used to say, leaning into me with a conspiratorial whisper, "If anything should happen to Winnie..." and how I'd thought the phrase a bizarre and peculiarly American euphemism. Surely "something" will happen to us all.

I dreamt that Peter and I were on vacation with our two children, a boy and a girl. I went ahead of them into a somehow tropical waiting room to buy coffee and hamburgers. I fumbled my change, which annoyed the woman behind the counter. We sat at a table in a plain white room where others were also waiting. There was a whoosh of sound and we looked out the windows to see the burning fuselage of a plane coming at us. No wings, just the bullet-shape with its windows aflame. Then it hit, searing a path through the undergrowth, and a wall of fire came through the café at us. We ran.

———

From Birgitt came a letter from one of their staff in Ethiopia, full of sadness, praising Tim for being "respectful and not just

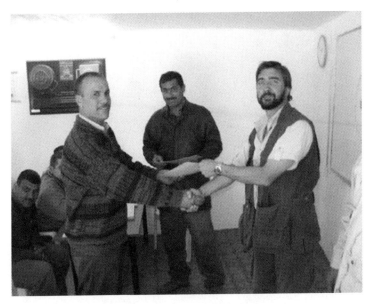

Graduation of the first 90 Iraqi de-miners, Baghdad, 2003.

like a boss"—and yet, Peter said, reminding him somehow of a letter of recommendation.

I said, "We don't know what's true any more."

He agreed. "Everything is PR—from grade inflation to celebrity to politics."

I said, *"Be all that you can be…"*

Also in that envelope, Birgitt had enclosed a DVD of an interview Tim did for Iraqi TV on the occasion of his team's graduation. I was afraid to watch it, then saw that I could not *not* watch it and loaded it onto the computer. The scene itself was familiar from stills Tim had copied onto my PC last January: a narrow whitewashed classroom, the ninety or so Iraqis at their desks, Tim at the front, bearded, casual in a many-pocketed khaki vest. There's a very brief interview in which he says bland things about how good his team is, then

Ambassador Patrick Kennedy speaks at greater bureaucratic length, at which it seems to me Tim's eyes slide ironic from side to side. Then the camera pans to a table on which are displayed types of explosive device. Tim's hand showing a mine. His face again.

Watching, I couldn't but put my hands out to touch him. But I was moved in a not unbearable, perhaps not even painful way, and I realized that it is easy for me to see him alive but almost impossible to see him dead. He is alive to me only in my memory but in my memory he can only be alive.

———

Back in Tallahassee I went to my GP to complain of my lethargy. I said I supposed it was depression, but she was luckily disinclined to diagnose any such thing as "all in my head." The blood work showed I'd had a case of mononucleosis—a teenager's disease!—which I'd already had at 21, and from which I'd supposed I was permanently protected. But apparently mono is one of those viruses that always lives on in the body, and in stress the immune system can be overwhelmed.

September. Hurricane Frances, for which we prepared with sandbags, batteries, and bottled water, merely soaked the inland panhandle in a long and dreary drizzle. I sat in my office watching mud flow down the patio, remembering the definition "dirt is matter out of place," and thinking that death, too, can be merely matter out of place. The pen with which I write this thought, no bigger around than a nine millimeter bullet, I manipulate over the paper, put in my pencil holder, drop on the floor, pick up again. It bodes no danger. But inserted the depth of a bullet into my brain, it would be as deadly.

On TV the third anniversary of 9/11 offered again and again—another-gain—the plane going into the second tower.

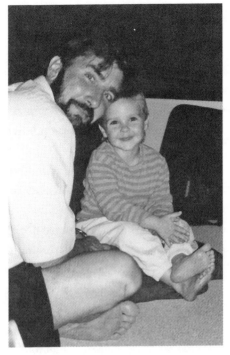

Tim and Thyra, Windhoek, Christmas 2003

I thought: *4/23 was my 9/11*, and then that the striking of the tower that I saw as it happened and have seen in rerun hundreds of times since, recurs in my mind the same way as the bullet going through Tim's brain, which I did not see. The same pattern, the same lethal penetration. Tearing its path. Always with the possibility that suicide is a form of terrorism: *See what you made me do.*

I think I understand (better now) how religion germinates in fear of the obliteration of a loved life. I glance up at Tim's picture—this one, say: cross-legged on the floor with Thyra, smiling straight at the camera, bronzed and bearded, the soles of his foot and her two feet at the same angle, the bottoms of their big toes white and tender-looking. The beloved dead still so exist in the synapses of our brains, how can they not have in fact, somewhere, at least that incorporeal life? *What, in the ground? What, dead? What is that?*

But I find no solace in the attempt to posit individual immortality. I understand that science is as much a myth as religion in the sense that its terms are made up by human beings to suit the workings of our own minds. But to suppose that the multifarious world can be—or only be!?—explained by "intelligent design" as our puny minds define it, is self-important, reductive, ignorant.

I must include these familiar musings because I am talking here about a soul precious to me and lost to me. The large question is: *how does physical matter make the quantum leap into subjective experience?* The answer is: *we don't know.* The question follows: *what happens when we die?* The answer: *we don't know.* Our guesses frighten us. *To sleep, perchance to dream. Ay, there's the rub.* But the preponderance of evidence is that when the physical entity degenerates, the psychic entity dissolves as well.

A year after Tim died I would start a long-planned novel. It was not autobiographical and had nothing to do with him. Nonetheless it was suddenly full of death and dying. *Dead child, dead child*: I gave my heroine a baby who lived less than a week, and I put her thoughts this way:

> *Nothing in her experience suggested that the personality would cohere beyond the body. On the contrary, recycling seemed the fundamental principle: nothing blooms but through decay. She believed only and absolutely in immortality at the subatomic level, and considered the nitrogen cycle sufficient marvel, sufficient glory.*

"*But that had not been put to the test, and now it was. Tentatively, and then fiercely, she embraced Chloe's dispersal into the universe. She lay awake at night allowing herself to contemplate the little body in its batiste dress in its maple coffin, welcoming the insects and the ooze, not flinching from the translucent larva, the self-generating maggots. She gathered this corruption in her arms and crooned to it. She held it to her heart. She lived the teeming, and then the subsiding, and then the still, ashen entropy of the beloved matter. Toenails, palms, iris, mole. Dust to dust. And then she slept.*

This *was* autobiographical, in a way I dared not then describe except through the scrim of fiction. I held Tim at night this way. For months. "Welcoming" is not wrong: I did not so much force as gently allow myself to see him in his grave, to picture what I know to be the mysterious process of corruption, as much a proof of the world's wonder as the process of animal birth. When I held him rotting was when I best understood the power of love.

8.

Six months on. I wanted, still, to sit staring into the beautiful baffle of trees outside my study window, raging if it took me that way, letting the tears well if I pleased, floating, disassociating on the intricate veining of the confederate ivy, which held each leaf open as the palm of a hand. Instead I inverted my own hands on what, for me, truly serve as keys; because this dogged syntax is how I unlock sense in the fleeting world. Because those who have tried to write honestly have helped me to make such sense.

———

When I left England and my husband in December of 1971, I brought the boys to my parents in Arizona for Christmas and then to Illinois, where my best friend, Julia Kling, lived with her husband, Blair. Though I was manic with freedom, somewhere in my subconscious I must have realized that I would need a friend.

I also brought us to poverty. I was pregnant, having conceived just as the marriage fell apart. Intimacy was by then so rare that I knew the date of the conception. I was prepared to have an abortion, but within a fortnight I miscarried. I got therapy. My parents bought me a $500 station wagon. I wrangled a teaching assistant's job at the University of Illinois and found a lucky sabbatical rental on a lake. I drank too much. I couldn't eat and became drastically thin. I suffered paroxysms of stage fright in the classroom. The money was so tight that we couldn't always manage a Saturday Dairy Queen. The need to get the boys on the school bus with their lunch money every morning seemed a monumental task, sometimes as much as I could manage in a day. When we later talked about that time, Tim and Alex protested that they'd assumed me competent and confident, whereas I felt I dragged myself from one precarious moment to the next. Even so I understood that I had good health, good kids, and the skill to make a living. I didn't see how any woman without those goods could function as a single mother.

In March, Walter flew from England to try for reconciliation, and a fellow novelist lent me her house so I had a place to retreat. One morning I found Tim at the breakfast table in tears. I asked what was wrong.

"Daddy wants me to help get you back and I don't know *how.*"

"That makes me very angry at Daddy," I said. "Of course you don't know how. It's not your job and it's not your problem."

I resolved then that I would never draw the children into our fight and would never say a word against their father—which was the right and even virtuous choice, although (I never met a motive I couldn't mix) I made it in prideful rage, and kept it with a sense of superiority.

It was harder to feel righteous when Walter demanded, "Why do *you* get to decide for all four of us?" I had no reply. I thought it was unfair too. But I felt that to go back to him would be defeat, possibly mortal, and this one constant in my mental chaos kept me headed into what looked like a bleak future. I knew Tim must blame me for the divorce, and there was a clear message to that effect when he made the purse-mouthed pronouncement: "You only get one chance at marriage." (He was twenty and back from a year living with his father before he said, "Mom, I never understood why you had to leave Daddy. Now I do.")

Between January and August the boys dropped their *jolly good*'s and took to saying *golly*. They fished in the lake, brought home good report cards and made friends in the neighborhood—Tim playing mostly cowboy while Toby at five declared himself a feminist and defended his right to play house. When I got a "real" job teaching lit and writing at Florida State, we moved down to Tallahassee, and Tim announced, seeing that their bedroom overlooked the apartment pool, "Oh, Mom, it's love at first sight!"

In Florida the boys swam, made friends, got camouflage outfits from the local Army Surplus, and joined war games in the swampy vacant lot next door. I continued rickety as a teacher, lonely and unstable in the evening hours, but I filed for divorce. I had by that time published three novels and was working on a fourth (about an awful marriage), and I wanted my maiden/professional name back as part of the divorce decree. There was no precedent for that in Florida. One day Toby/Alex came home in a tearful tantrum because the first-grade teacher had taken his class to show them how to use the library, and he had checked out *The Giant Jam Sandwich*, boasting that his mother was the author.

The teacher said, "*Now*, Toby..."

He demanded, spluttering, "You tell her, you write a note...!"

My lawyer fastened on this as proof that retaining my husband's name could in fact harm my boys. Relishing the opportunity to set a feminist precedent, he used the incident to get Burroway back without my having to file a separate claim.

Like many people and most writers (also saints and schizophrenics), I have a symbolic turn of mind, and this was no doubt transferred for good and ill to both my sons. When Tobyn was born, my mother wrote asking whether I realized that the middle initial of my grandfather, Dana T. Milner, was Tobin, his mother's maiden name—"though he hated the Tobins, and always pretended that his middle initial stood for *Timothy*."

This had just the right combination of coincidence, subconsciousness, and wonder for me. I supposed that as a child I must have heard this tale and somehow dredged it up to name two sons for my beloved grandfather. Later, though, the younger of them may have realized that his nickname was popular for British dogs and the "Toby jug," a low-end tourist trinket named for a Shakespearean fat man. By the time he was eight his brother was tall, thin, cool, and "a brain"—the desirables of middle school. Toby, plump, a natural rebel, wore his envy in such a way that if someone praised his thick eyelashes, he translated, "They mean I'm fat."

One day he came to me: "Mom, *Toby* is a kind of *round* name, isn't it?"

"Why, yes, that's very clever."

"*Tim* is a straight up-and-down name."

"I guess it is."

"From now on my name is Alex."

And *Alex* is how he remade himself, eventually outstripping Tim in height, taking up acting, the guitar, and computer games, excelling in "gifted" classes while he persistently got Ds in math and artistically shredded his sleeves. For two years after his announcement of the name change, he patiently or impatiently corrected me every time I called him Toby.

Whether in his transformation Alex remembered that I had fought legally for Burroway I don't know. Nor do I know whether Tim suffered from the difference in our last names.

He seemed to me absolutely adjusted until I began to date. Then one evening when I ventured out to a party with a friend (not a sexual partner and not a romance), Tim scowled, "I don't want Vaughn to be my father!"

I drew him up short. "Vaughn isn't going to be your father. You *have* a father. And we're not getting married, we're going to Maxine's."

But the next year, when I *was* dating and Walter was headed for a second marriage, Tim's suffering surfaced. He came out one afternoon from the bedroom where I had set up bunks in an on-the-cheap attempt to reproduce their Sussex room. His hair fell sun-bleached across his forehead, his cheeks blanched. I was dressing for a date, hooking my earrings in. "I like John," he said, "but..." His face screwed up, and it was then he explained "pungee sticks," which John, who had been a radio operator in Vietnam, had told him about. A whittled branch is smeared with dog shit; if you don't die of the wound you die of infection. Tim said, "I sit in school feeling my insides scrape. If I knew how to go on scraping, I could kill myself that way." I was shocked. I stayed home. But in its context of days it was an exceptional moment, and I saw my job as simply to reassure him every way I could that his father and I both loved him and that divorce did not touch that fact. Seven years later I would take Alex to a counselor for no more reason than that we were getting on each other's nerves. In 1974 it neither occurred to me to "get Tim help," nor do I think he would have agreed to it.

Their father remarried, and Toby/Alex took his usual upbeat view of things, boasting that he had *two* mothers. Tim came back from vacation in their new Minnesota home much mollified, impressed with his stepmother, Barbi, who had an unfailing sense of style, and who (again, the boys

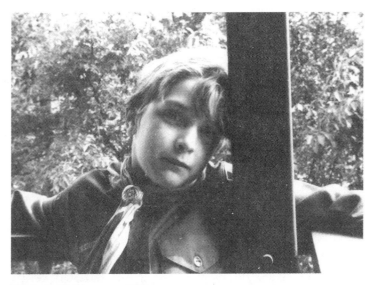

The Scout, Tallahassee, c. 1976

voiced this years later) was "much better than you were at handling Daddy."

"She just lets him rant," one of them—I think it was Alex—said, "and then she says, *Oh, Walter.*"

Growing up in Florida, Tim was modest, intense, and fiercely honorable, and he had few but deep friendships. He lit with enthusiasm for his most demanding teachers, praising their strictness, their discipline. He was from the beginning a worrier after his own integrity, which he pursued with solemn doggedness. Once, after we had moved from the apartment to a concrete-block bungalow, the boys discovered a cache of professional archery equipment, still in its original carton in a hollow log in a nearby woods. The label bore an address to a local sporting goods shop. Alex and I admired the glossy laminated woods, and wavered, tempted. But Tim was adamant: we had to drive to the shop to return it *right now*. It turned out that the equipment had been stolen from a city park recreation center. I was somewhat sheepish in the face of my son's virtue, and annoyed that neither the shop nor the city acknowledged his honesty, for which, however, Tim seemed to need no reward.

There was another day that he came home from middle school with a detention slip. He'd been called into the principal's office for "bad language," and the principal asked if his mother knew he used those words. Tim said a little defiantly that she did. The principal then asked if his mother *approved* of those words. Tim knew perfectly well that as far as I was concerned, "bad language" is mendacious, ungrammatical, or inexact, and that swearing is sometimes the optimal way to say a thing. It still raises my ire that a professional educator would put a boy in this dilemma, having to choose between a lie and a slur on his mother. It's a small template of his priorities that this particular boy, with his moralist's code and his cherry tree for bones, hesitated and then said, "No, sir, she does not approve."

Sometimes he did not approve of me. He liked me in suits, not sundresses. When the new puppy crapped on the doormat, he told me I "kept an unsanitary house." (I handed him the soap and brush.) When I bought a Honda Civic he said he preferred to "see me in something more upscale."

In 1975 I sold the novel *Raw Silk* for both publication and magazine condensation, dared a bigger mortgage, and we moved across town to a thirties white-brick house with the look of an English cottage. It was airy and spacious and full of avocado shag that I would vanquish room by room; and a finished attic with two slope-roofed bedrooms, for which Alex chose a wild-animal motif while Tim painted his red, white, and blue, and I made him a quilt of denim stars and stripes. This house had a fenced dog yard for hound-mutt Shirley, a bank of azaleas that rioted every February, and an acre of its own woods—a canopy of live oak, magnolia, camphor, tung, and pines ninety feet above our heads. I hired a student to help build a treehouse anchored on three water oaks—which Tim and Alex furnished with jetsam and paraphernalia of their own invention.

In the rec room of the De Soto St. house was a hanging lamp on a pulley to adjust its height. A couple of times when I reached up to turn it on I got a shock and made a mental note that it ought to be replaced. It didn't register as important. One evening I was entertaining friends, Tim holding forth to them on some subject of preteen urgency. He had one hand on the refrigerator just beyond the kitchen arch, and with the other idly reached up to pull down the lamp. He stopped mid-sentence, and began to bend slowly, slowly back, as if doing a backbend. Somebody giggled, thinking he was clowning. I knew slapstick sight gags were not his style. I lurched toward him. Luckily the fuse blew before I got there, for I would merely have extended the conduction. He fell back on the floor, me on top of him. He shook and babbled and complained of cold. We put him to bed in my room and loaded him with blankets. "Get rid of that lamp!" he said. I said I would. Later, when he had calmed, he said, "My head was surrounded with jagged black and red lines, like in a cartoon."

Could this have damaged or rewired some synapses in his brain? No. Silly. Once backstage as a girl I took hold of a live wire. Once Peter as a boy was tricked into climbing an electrified statue. No—but the visceral power of memory is such that, writing of this close call now, my heart is pounding with fear for a life already lost.

———

Tim's relationship with his father continued problematic. Tim had, for instance, a battalion or two of the kind of plastic soldiers that come forty to a pack. He painted them, positioned them, built tanks for them and arranged elaborate dioramas. Once when he was at his father's house, Walter "caught him" chopping off half a dozen plastic arms and legs. Walter flew into a rage, accusing him of vicarious torture and mutilation. Tim called me hot with the injustice of it. "I wouldn't! They only come in four positions. I just wanted to have more ways they could stand and hold their guns and stuff."

When Tim was headed into high school, Walter proposed that he should spend a semester in Pittsburgh. Tim wanted to try it. I agreed, but said he should know he could come back to Tallahassee any time he chose. Tim said, "I think it's time I learned to stand up to my dad."

I remember one phone call a few months later after which Alex found me in tears because, I told him, I'd heard in Tim's voice that he was going to stay up there. Tim came home for the summer with the question not decided. One evening driving him to his speed-skating team, I said, "You may not realize this, but you're under pressure because whatever choice you make, it'll be an implied rejection of the other parent."

Tim said, "*Boy*, do I realize that!"

My memory makes it the next afternoon that I heard Tim on the phone with his father. "No, Dad." And then a silence. "No, but…No, Dad…but Mom doesn't put me under pressure like you do." He held the phone away from his ear and I could hear the shouting from across the room. Tim listened in silence, looked at the receiver and gently put it down.

"He hung up on me."

I nodded. "You were the adult in that exchange."

He stayed in Tallahassee.

———

When I look back on those years, my own regrets are not of my permissiveness toward the children, which in most ways I think did them good, but that I permitted myself the serial monogamy of the zeitgeist.

The years between 1965 and 1975, which now prompt a general launching of rotten eggs, seem to me in many ways superior to our current era—tolerant, open to ideas, compassionate to the poor, energetic for social change. Sexual liberation, on the other hand, seduced a lot of us into a dreary round. The pressure toward chastity of my childhood turned a hundred and eighty degrees toward a pressure for sexual free-spiritedness—and the one led to about as much deceit and self-deception as the other. A character in one of my plays says, "I think there's a lot more celibacy going on than people are generally willing to admit." There was also, even at the height of the women's movement, a lot of flailing about to find Mr. Right.

I had a four-year second marriage to a young artist, funny and kind, who was however eighteen years younger than I and therefore never a serious candidate for permanence. (I did not see this, of course.) Otherwise I fell into a pattern, which you could say was later repeated by Tim, of romances that would last two or three years and then dwindle to a sometimes-more, sometimes-less amiable demise.

The brother of one of these boyfriends was a recreation-parachutist who two or three times took the boys up to watch him jump, instilling in Tim (not Alex) an ambition to do the same. This brother later bamboozled an insurance company and was eventually jailed in New York for passing counterfeit twenties he had printed not far from our house. When—with a little trepidation, because Tim liked the man, and I knew he would be shocked—I told Tim of the arrest, Tim said, "I don't think he did it for the money. It was because he liked the risk."

Tim was then perhaps eleven. I thought it an insight beyond his years. I did not see that "liking risk" might have been a projection of his own predilection.

——

"Loneliness," says Anne Carson, "is not an important form of suffering. It's undeniable, but it's just not significant." I wish I had encountered that opinion in the seventies, and having encountered it could have believed it. Once on a panel of writers I heard myself saying, "I decided to be a writer when I was about seventeen, and I have never since made a major life decision in the service of my writing." I was startled at the truth I'd blurted out. In later years of male "reconstruction" I frequently ran across a dictum such as, "No man ever looked back over his life wishing he'd spent more time in the office." Maybe, but if I had it to do over again, I'd endure fewer parties and partners and spend more Saturday nights learning Farsi and astronomy.

Shortly after my second marriage ended I met Rob Jones, a former Green Beret who'd come to FSU for his Ph.D. in English—*rebound* might come to mind. In any case I was vulnerable and he was protective. He was divorced, the father of three, courtly in the extreme, generous to the edge of oppressive, and romantic in a markedly door-opening Victorian way. He was also a decorated Vietnam veteran of at least two tours, an outspoken scold of the liberal left, and a lover of all things warlike. He had the requisite T-shirt that said, "Kill 'em all. Let God sort 'em out." His cottage on Lake

Talquin, described by one of my male colleagues as "every boy's dream," contained an extensive collection of guns, knives, military paraphernalia, and expensive tweed that was gradually being demolished by the moths and mildew of the Florida panhandle. When he wanted to give a party, Rob shot a few squirrels, skinned them, and boiled up a stew.

My friends were quick to opine that the major was a major mismatch for me, but Tim, then in high school, took to and ultimately idolized him; and there grew between them a bond that was partly born of being two warrior-hunters in a liberal university milieu, but also I think a deeper accord. Both felt they had been born a century too late. Both yearned for the test of their mettle. Rob had been shrapnel-wounded several times and used to boast, "The trick is not minding that it hurts." Tim took this particular brand of toughness as a touchstone. Later in Ranger School, humping a hundred and twenty pounds over a mountain trail without sleep or food for forty hours, he would use it as an under-the-breath marching song: The *trick* is not *mind*ing that it *hurts*. The *trick*...

Rob was a heavy drinker of the good-natured sort that transactional analyst Claude Steiner calls the "Drunk and Proud." I could hold my liquor pretty well myself, and this is probably the place to say that it was during the period I dated Rob that I faced (as I had long denied) that this was not a good thing, and that I had already downed my share of the world's alcohol. I had grown up in a Methodist household of such righteous abstention that my mother boasted there'd never been an ashtray or a wine glass on the premises—so when I went to New York at nineteen the particular fetish of my rebellion was already chosen. I had drunk "socially" until my marriage to Walter unraveled and had "self-medicated" after that (I'm not sure these designations are distinct). In the lonely marital aftermath I solaced myself with the Bourbon brothers George, Jack, and Jim. Being with Rob only clarified how I drank: steadily, excessively, and unlike him with crushing guilt. While he was on Reserve duty in Norfolk I joined a recovery group. As soon as I was pretty certain my sobriety would take, I told the boys about it, to their mutual amazement.

I remember balancing on the unstable edge of the rec-room couch, Tim loafer-shod and Izod-shirted in an easy chair, Alex on the floor, rail-skinny by now, ear-pierced and pre-punk in a T-shirt with the sleeves torn out. I rarely assembled them outside of dinnertime, so there was an air of apprehension. I explained that it made me uneasy to lie about where I went every evening, when the whole point was getting honest. So I thought it was time to let them in on what I was doing.

Tim said, "I know a lot of people I think are alcoholics, Mom, but you were *not* on my list."

Alex said, "Are you *sure?* That means we've got the gene both sides."

I agreed. "You'll have to be careful."

They were not the only ones who thought I melodramatized. My friend Mari said, "Oh, for heaven's sake, why can't you just drink too much? Why do you have to be an alcoholic?" Rob said, "If you think you need to cut down, do it. You don't need that fuzzy stuff."

Members of the recovery group, though, recognized me as a "high-bottom"—meaning that I had acknowledged my problem ("hit bottom") before it cost me a job, a family, an accident, or jail time, but that I was inexorably headed down that alley. "High-bottom" is a form of the disease common to achieving women, those of us who are trained and adept at smoothing feathers, keeping things together. I had come to feel, in these womanly tasks—and in the classroom, where I often felt I was "pretending to teach"—that I was standing in the middle of a life-lie. Sobriety righted me, and though that is another story, it's fair to say that I when I turned away from alcohol I turned toward work and love, both of which together made happiness possible for me. Much later, after Tim and Birgitt were married, I was startled to learn that Tim had not admitted my alcoholism to Birgitt. He had told her I "didn't drink," protecting my reputation as he had with the middle-school principal. Which also means of course that he was ashamed.

It may be that, just as Tim's need of his father had kept me in that marriage, his reverence for Rob kept me in the affair past its sell-by date. It may be that Rob's influence pushed Tim farther in the bellicose direction he was already headed. It may be that Tim's foundering relationship with his father was further damaged by the contrast with this soldier and his unconditional machismo. All that may be. It's also the case that Tim found in Rob something he had sought and lacked, and that Rob accepted him as a son long after our infirm affair had ended. After Tim's death I found two yearning mentions of Rob among his freshman college essays. In one he hoped that "maybe with luck we will be" a family. The other eulogizes the Rob-figure as a hero who deftly disarms a mugger, whose "views are slightly right, but keeps an open mind," who "believes in America, something not often seen in people these days," and who "is not my biological father, but the father of my spirit."

As he came through puberty Tim read voraciously, mostly adventure novels, admired John Wayne's acting and his politics, and more than once to my despair quoted, "My country, right or wrong." At eighteen he came home at three one morning, in tears because he could not go to defend England's honor in the Falklands. Shortly thereafter I realized that both my boys, who had spent their early years in shoulder-length dirty-blond shag, had shaved their heads—Alex for a Mohawk and Tim for ROTC. Both wore combat boots, the one for busking around the Eros statue in London, the other for jumping out of airplanes. It occurred to me that Tim was rebelling against sixties parents, the ones who had him out in the stroller at the sit-ins or confined to his playpen while we addressed envelopes for Mother Against the Bomb. Alex, instead of rebelling against Mom (what's the point?—if she'll let you be a soldier, she'll let you be anything), rebelled against his big brother, the hero-worship and the Top Siders, all things buttondown or flag-waving.

Much of the time it seemed funny, and when we fought, my battles with Alex were the more bitter precisely because he and I were more alike. His impulses were generous, sloppy, and full of turmoil, whereas Tim would hold back and calmly stand his ground. Alex was a loud and messy liberal, like me. Tim said "Yes, ma'am," ready to do a task right now, and I had to be grateful for military virtues in a son.

Nevertheless, when I disagreed with Tim there was a higher proportion of subtext to text. Our quarrels were less frequent and less personal, but they betrayed a deeper divide. I remember one evening in a slightly stuffy, pleasantly scruffy London flat with worn leather on the chairs, Kurdish rugs on the floor, and middle-aged versions of the Cambridge undergraduates we had mostly been—now pundits, publishers, writers, and actors, what the British call the "chattering classes." Both my sons were with me on this trip, sixteen-year-old Alex out with his guitar and the punks of Piccadilly

Circus, nineteen-year-old Tim somewhere in the adjoining room in Harris tweed. I recognized the man crossing toward me, glass in hand, as somebody I vaguely knew—first name Jeff (or Geoff), last name lost. Slender, sandy, he looked too young to be the president of London PEN International, though I seemed to remember that's what he was. I remembered he was witty and articulate, an impassioned campaigner for the freeing of imprisoned writers; my kind of person. So I was glad to see him headed toward me.

He charged a little purposefully, though, his look a little heated. "I've been talking to your son," he said, and set his glass against his chin. "My God, how do you stand it?!"

My stomach clenched around its undigested canapés, brain wrung like a sponge. Shame, defensiveness, and rage (*I am responsible for my son; I am not responsible for my son; who are you to insult my son?*) so filled my throat that I could not immediately speak. What I felt was that I, literally, closed down. The free-speech champion offered me the kind of face, sympathy and shock compounded, that one offers to the victim of mortal news.

"I manage," I managed presently, and turned on my heel.

I have never so far as I know run into Jeff or Geoff again, but I credit him with the defining moment, when choice is made at depth: the Mother Moment.

9.

In October, Peter and I drove to visit his family in Milwaukee, in November flew to see my brother Stan and his wife, Liz, in Reno. I realized that we were performing a natural ritual by touching down at extended family. When I made some reference to Tim's life having been cut short, my brother said, "Every life is complete. Some are short stories and some are epics, but every one is whole." This was comfort. He said, "We'll never know how many children will maintain all four of their limbs because Tim did the work he did."

Back in Tallahassee we held our traditional Thanksgiving dinner for a couple of dozen. I made the gravy that everyone remembered had been Tim's job when he was home. "He always used too much thyme," I pointed out, and they laughed, agreeing.

We managed Christmas with a modicum of the usual fuss and fun, and then on the other side of the world the tsunami came, literally flooding more families with more sorrow than I could contain in my imagination: twenty-three thousand dead, thirty, thirty-three. I remembered the film *Hiroshima, Mon Amour*, and what I always took to be its theme: that catastrophe can only be experienced one person at a time.

My tsunami. Gun and gone. Forever. What is dead?

I went up the woods path to the swing, could not sit still, walked back through the trees howling, trying to do it on my own, not always to take it to Peter. But could not. And he (always): "I want you to bring it to me. I want to help."

Later he summed up the year: "2004. Mistakes were made."

———

There were always new ways I could be flung back into mourning, and many were trivial, undignified. The sight of women with small boys would make me hunch over my supermarket cart and turn into an empty aisle. The mail came relentlessly addressed to Tim, catalogues of guns, offers of credit, clothing sales. Once I addressed an email to Alex by mistake to Tim's old address, and got it back marked "permanent fatal error."

Then those days of January 2005 came around that were the first of the anniversaries: *a year since the last time I saw him alive.* On the 24th of February he would have been forty-one. *Except, he will be forty forever.*

"No," Joyce said gently, "forty is not what he will be."

On the back deck at home the scuppernong vine came into leaf and stretched to the far corners of the pergola. The tendrils caught at every nail or splinter. The leaves, translucent at first, unfurled in their hundreds. Three or four times a day I walked under them, thinking with Robert Frost that spring announces itself not in green but in gold. It was Peter who had planted and tended this vine, but its burgeoning seemed to embody birth, warmth, the urge to grow—almost unbearable in its evocation. First anniversary of Casey Sheehan's death. First anniversary of Pat Tillman's. It was a matter of wonder to me that there had already lived on earth someone who had said, "April is the cruelest month." What was I to make of the fact that Tim died on Shakespeare's birthday? Nothing. Silly coincidence. But how, in any case, had I come to know so many lines about a single month?

"Whan that Aprill with his shoures soote…"

"On the eighteenth of April, in Seventy-five;
Hardly a man is now alive…"

"Men are April when they woo…"

"Oh, to be in England now that April's there…"

"On the side of a hill
In the month of April
I was with her
In beautiful weather."

"…the sweet small clumsy feet of April came…"

For the weekend that included April 23rd, the first anniversary of Tim's death, we rented a beach house with old friends. Eight of us, including seven- and nine-year-old Phoebe and Flannery Stuckey-French, drove to St. George Island on the Gulf and spread our gear over the sofas and porches of a glorious villa, stucco on stilts, with picture windows onto the dunes and the sea. The weather was balmy, the sea oats waving, the sand white grit between our toes. The girls squealed for Peter to tell them ghost stories, and we gorged on shrimp and scallops and pistachios. The TV kept up a steady background of NBA. Serious Scrabble tournaments occurred. I may even have played Monopoly with the girls.

Here, the pelicans plummeting into the surf, the dolphins arching twenty yards offshore, I kept Tim cocooned in my consciousness, just gently with me. I fell into a predictable pattern, although I did not predict it: I got through the difficult anniversary just fine, and then the next day, drying myself in front of an unfamiliar mirror in unfamiliar light, I noticed under my breast and down my side a sprinkling of flat red moles, perhaps five of them, with a bluish cast. My doctor had pointed these out—when was that, October?—had measured them in millimeters and told me to keep an eye on them. I had forgotten this. They were still no larger than small sequins, which they somewhat resembled. But they had clearly grown.

I couldn't get an appointment for a week. In the meantime I must fly to New Hampshire to direct a review of the Dartmouth Creative Writing Program. And the pattern continued. As long as I was concentrating and engaged, enjoying the people, the work, and the graceful campus, I recognized myself, me-getting-on-with-it. But on the bus ride back to the airport through the bleak still-bare forests (four days ago I'd been barefoot in lapping surf), I was taken out of the self I knew and set naked into the space occupied by universal winter. I was "beside myself." I was sixty-eight; my mother had died at sixty-eight. Tim had chosen to die a year ago. I was not now in the forward path of my expectation, but allied to the dead, drawn toward them by an undertow that registered dragging in my body as the bus heaved itself over another rise. And in the midst of this supposed apocalypse my efficient mind began its works—divvying up the china, devolving the flat to Alex, cleansing the computer.

It was nonsense. My GP and then a dermatologist confirmed that these were harmless age spots, not the reaper's signature on my dance card. I laugh at myself. I see the nature of the repetition: a trial courageously passed, followed by a foolishness, followed by identification with the dead. It is, perhaps, a kind of practice. One of my heroines says, "The old are not hypochondriacal, they are *prescient*. This slicing at the ribs is heart attack, though perhaps not now. This swelling in the lymph nodes is cancer, just perhaps not here." When, later, I encountered Thomas Joiner's theory that serious candidates for suicide inure themselves to pain and danger, I thought that perhaps one purpose of the piecemeal decline of the human body is, more generally, to habituate us to our own demise.

———

Now began the litigation that would bring Birgitt, Thyra, and eventually Neal to America, and would absorb Birgitt's energy for half a dozen years. Convinced that Tim had suffered from PTSD, Birgitt sought out Gary Pitts, a Houston-based lawyer specializing in DBA, or "The Defense Base Act Extension of the Longshore and Harbor Workers' Compensation Act." This law propounded that if a person died as a result of work done under contract to the U.S. government, the spouse and children deserved some benefits. Pitts would try to show that Tim's "exposure to 'the zone of special danger' in Iraq aggravated or accelerated his preexisting psychic condition to the point that he committed suicide." Lawyers for RONCO, or rather for their insurance company Continental Casualty, would argue otherwise.

Birgitt gathered for exhibit Tim's emails, Army reports, photographs, statements of friends—evidence on the one hand of the normality of their family life and, on the other, of the dangers Tim had faced in Iraq and the anomalies in his behavior when he returned.

She also received, from Rob Jones, at least one foreshadowing of the resistance she would encounter to a diagnosis of PTSD.

The major's email covered four single-spaced pages of

impassioned "defense" of Tim that downplayed both the stresses of the de-mining job and the impact of Tim's disillusionment. Rob was "appalled and horrified to see Tim so dismissed and trivialized by this perverse interpretation of his life," which in Rob's view was no more than a cover for "snivelers and whiners." He wrote:

> *"The simple reality is that he was not . . . in a life-threatening environment . . . not witness to extended horrors of the battleground . . . not afraid for his life beyond any normal human response to an environment where violence is ongoing . . . "*

Rob argued that Tim went into de-mining operations "because he rejected other options that were boring and meaningless to him" and not because he was "dedicated to any silly crusade against landmines."

I was moved by the headlong rush of Rob's letter, which these quotations scarcely convey, and which spoke of his love for my son at the far reaches of his personality, where I could not follow, to which I was alien. I found the letter breathtaking in both its force and its reasoning, so topsy-turvy to my own—mine being a sort of reasoning Rob dismissed as coming from a "small coterie of academics, aging holdovers from the sixties and seventies . . ."

Got me there.

I tried to balance these two Tims in my mind: both honorable, both patriotic, both drawn to danger—Rob's Tim a realistic administrator making a mature choice of the less humdrum job, mine an idealistic man/boy who longed to see things with the moral certainty of the warrior—but could not. I remember once saying to Rob after he had told some

Vietnam story, "It must be comfortable to know who the enemy is." He had agreed without irony that it was.

––––––

Birgitt carried on in the moral certainty that she was "defending Tim's honor" by the very diagnosis that Rob thought humiliated him. If Tim had "snapped," she reasoned, he was not responsible for his suicide. Nor was she. I pointed out that if she claimed too perfect a marriage she undercut her own case, since marital friction was a known sign of post-traumatic stress.

Distant from both Rob's view and Birgitt's, ambivalent about intruding the law into my fragile recovery, I nevertheless agreed to be deposed by phone and witness at the trial. But I knew that my memories of Tim came in disconnected scenes and sequence, so Peter and I sat down to reconstruct a chronology of Tim's adult life with the help of letters, photo albums, and the daily calendars I'd obsessively squirreled away. Too often these said "Call Tim" without indicating in what hemisphere to call him, or "Tim back from Ghana" when "back" meant back to Germany or Cameroon. Sometimes his comings and goings crisscrossed ours to Florence, London, Budapest. Sometimes both boys were home for Christmas, other years only one, or neither. Peter and I each had memory markers—that birthday at Pelican Roost with Jewel, the time Tim brought Anne the pogo stick—was that the same summer the hophead crashed into the Prelude? Peter tended to remember cars and meals; I retained scraps of talk and holidays.

I did not know, and do not, whether Tim had PTSD. I learned from his Reserve officer's assessment that he was "sole contingency operations planner" for a "rescue recovery

attempt" after the collision of American and German heli-
copters off the coast of Namibia—and that "attempt" implies
dead bodies. I know from Birgitt that he saw American soldiers shooting unprovoked into Iraqi houses and that he
thought his plane was being attacked by missiles as he left
Iraq. I don't know whether these amounted to trauma or
"merely" contributed to life-denying depression. This project
did not help me to know. And yet laying out the facts also laid
bare the central pattern of Tim's life, an abiding need for family and the pull of adventure, a conflict between belonging
and solitude—and his awkward, touching attempts somehow
to reconcile them.

I wouldn't make too much of his first high-school girlfriend being a majorette in a marching band, but each of the
young women who later caught his heart had in some way
an exotic background, or at least ancestry other than American mainland. Nathalie he found in college ROTC, who had
been adopted by an American Army officer as an infant from
a Vietnamese orphanage, and who herself contained the contradiction of delicate Asian features, a raucous laugh, and a
Floridian sweep of gesture. Linda was Haole, with whom
Tim lived briefly when he was stationed in Hawaii. Despina
was Greek, her father a manufacturer in Cameroon. Jewel's
tradition-sensitive family was Indian Sikh transplanted to
Tallahassee. Birgitt was a "white African" in the problematic
term. In each of these relationships there had occurred some
crisis of commitment, followed by a retreat into the warrior-
hunter life.

Tim had been gawky in his teens, shag-haired and rab-
bit-toothed before his mouth was reined in by braces, even
while his little brother shot up past him in height and self-
assuredness. But in his mid-twenties Tim woke up one day

a handsome man. He had his father's thick wavy hair and powerful voice, my father's blue eyes, my jaw, his posture from calisthenics; not tall—he was stretching it to call himself 5'10"—but well proportioned and forceful. He had his father's attention to sartorial detail but better taste in ties and tweed. Like his father he evolved into a superb cook (and like his father left the kitchen a bomb site). When he broke his nose in "a stupid ROTC game" and it failed to set aright, I drove to Gainesville and stayed while he underwent plastic surgery. He'd been born with his father's Roman proboscis, and the surgeon offered "while he was at it" to straighten out the bend. Undecided to the very last minute, Tim agreed, with the result that his profile was handsomer than either his father's or mine, though I think he always had doubts, as of filial disloyalty.

When they were children both Tim and Alex took pride in hearing family legends, that we were related to Louisa May Alcott on my mother's side, and especially that, as descendants of my paternal grandmother, they could claim membership in the McKenzie clan of Scotland. They divided neatly, though, over their choice of McKenzie mottos. Alex picked the Latin *luceo non uro,* "Light not heat," while Tim hewed to the Gaelic that translated "All for the king!"

From boyhood (do I mean "always," or only "after the divorce"?), Tim evinced a respect both sentimental and profound for the idea of family. The siblings of his father's second marriage were never "half-" but fully acknowledged as brother and sister. Peter's daughter Anne was not *step-* but *sister,* and eventually he would insist that Neal was his *son.*

In the 1990s Tim's father's family moved to Cairo, where Walter ran the theatre department of the American University. Tim visited them there from Cameroon and

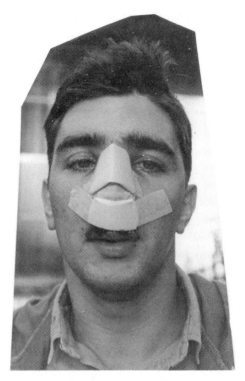

Nose job; Gainesville, Florida, 1984

found himself defending his teenaged half-brother against condemnations that were familiar in tone if not in content. Tim began to say, as would over the years become a mantra, "What I've learned from my father is how not to be a father." At the same time his respect for his stepmother, Barbi, intensified. He reported with approval that she'd admitted her life was difficult, but that she'd made a conscious decision to stay in the marriage for the children's sake. This he told me in a warmly confidential way, no sting apparently intended, so that I don't know even now whether he was aware of comparing her to me.

All these, even his judgment of his father, were evidence of his hot defense of family. But for himself, faced with a woman's expectation of commitment, Tim was likely to flee—even literally to fly away.

———

Tim and Jewel met during a Christmas vacation in Tallahassee, at just about the same time Peter and I got together. Peter was a colleague in modern languages in the building next to mine on the Florida State campus, and he and his former wife and I had been members of the same social group for eighteen years. This meant evenings arguing German expressionist film or deconstruction as well as shared beach vacations, Thanksgiving dinners, and Christmas parties. Consequently Tim had known the Rupperts for more than half his life. He later loved to tell how, one Thanksgiving when he was at the stove stirring the famous thyme gravy, I sat with one-year-old Anne Ruppert on my knee, teasing him. "Tim, don't you want to bring me one of these?" Nothing was then further from either of our minds than that this infant would become my stepdaughter, a decade in advance of Tim's bringing home a grandchild.

I had always liked the Rupperts but been not particularly close to either, had always thought Peter handsome but never given him a romantic thought (I didn't do husbands), and was later grateful that I was in England the year their marriage came apart. After they separated Peter and I began taking in films and food together, and by late 1991 when Tim left the Army we were, as we called it, "living together in two houses."

So we two couples saw a lot of each other that year of Tim's unhappy Dean Witter-ing. He and Jewel were in love with a mutual wide-eyed yearning, but the problem surfaced that was never solved. He wanted out of a suit and tie and into world adventure. She did not want to tag along. She was then working as a counselor in Social Security, was good at it, and was supremely employable. She would, she said, go with him anywhere in the United States and find work wherever they touched down. But she wouldn't be a soldier's wife, mercenary or otherwise.

Then Rob Jones offered Tim Africa, and in 1992 he went, one eye over his shoulder, to Yaounde, Cameroon, to train guards for the embassies and multinational corporations. When he had leave enough, he would fly back to Tallahassee, trying to convince Jewel to join him, at least to visit Cameroon. But why would she join him where she feared West African bigotry against East Indians?

Meanwhile, working with Rob and later on his own, Tim traveled around Africa for the Wackenhut Company, an outfit out of Miami that had been started by four ex-FBI agents and had now become one of the largest private security companies in the world. He helped set up training programs in Sierra Leone, Liberia, and the Ivory Coast. He took up horseback riding and acquired passable French, sent for Peter's homegrown jalapeños and introduced Mexican cooking to Yaounde.

He joined the Army reserve, and because he did this while in Africa, his home base was Stuttgart, from where he volunteered for everything in sight, was in subsequent years sent to Sarajevo and then the Republic of Congo, where, he told me, he was conscious of "making a difference" and "being on the tip of the spear." In those days I wrote of him that he was "a computer whiz with the soul of a Musketeer" and that I was forced to be aware of my own contradictions in his presence:

a feminist often charmed by his machismo, a pacifist with a temper, an ironist moved by his rhetoric.

His longest letters detailed the hunting trips (and, meaningless to me, the guns he used) in Garoua and into the bush at Buffle Noir, bargaining for cash and meat with guides and porters, stalking eland, bubale (haartebeest), hippotrague (roan antelope), and warthog. A handwritten note on the back of one of these letters says that Jewel found his trophy photos disgusting. She wanted to save the picture of him and cut the dead animals away. This, he said, was "a major problem" and "is certainly indicative of a desire for a different lifestyle. Would appreciate your comments on this"—which for all its stilted syntax was rather bold of him, since he surely knew I would side with Jewel and the haartebeest.

———

After a cancer struggle of several years' duration, in October of 1995, Walter died. Both boys had visited his sickbed in Belgium, and even so his death took both by surprise. Each of them called me. Each was stressed, anecdotal, somewhat bewildered. Each separately said, "I always thought I'd have a chance to get to know my father."

It was May of the next year that Alex called to announce that Tricia was pregnant. What's more, she was five months along, which meant that Peter and I, scheduled to teach on the fall FSU London Program, would be there when the baby was born.

"Tell Tim I win," Alex said.

At the pool where Tim was sunning with his nose in a Tom Clancy or Wilbur Smith, I passed on the taunt. Tim gave a good-natured grin. "I was just thinking the same thing."

In fact, when Eleanor was born in September, Tim was

back in Europe on Reserve assignment and so was able to cross to England to see his niece just a few days old. Alex clowned proud-Papa for my camera in front of a "House of Toby" ale sign, and Peter and the brothers drank a pint to Eleanor while Tim spread out his snapshots of Sarajevo, the pale ancient walls, the conical towers, himself on a bridge in camouflage with a rifle slung from one shoulder.

Looking back I see in those sets of photos—a newborn on the one hand, an automatic rifle on the other—ample sign of the gulf between them. But it is also true that the baby brought out an awestruck tenderness in Tim, and for that charged weekend what registered between the brothers was mutual warmth and mutual pride.

10.

Through the nineties Tim's interest in guns persisted and increased. *Interest* and *persisted* and *increased* are neutral words, the rhetoric of fact. What they leave out is the mother-son dance of discomfort, denial, acceptance, effort, defensiveness, rupture, affection, *politesse*. Tim never failed to bring and show off a new acquisition. He would lay a rifle across my hands with a grin of expectant pride. I would nod and weigh it and hum in the back of my throat and hand it back. I think on his part there remained a belief that if he could once convince me of the beauty of this wood grain, the miraculous action of this bolt, I would see the nobility of his infatuation. For my part I held the rose-tinted hope that, as with speed skating or scuba diving, which had also needed expensive state-of-the-art gear, if I just kept my counsel the fad would pass.

And yet I sometimes saw, well enough to put in words, that "this is who he is, and has been consistently from babyhood," or that he might spend "several hundred hours filing every edge inside and out so that all the parts fit with silken smoothness" in the same way as I "worry my lines across the page one at a time, take apart and refit the housing of the sentences, polish and shine."

But how should I persuade myself that my son loved weapons the way I love language? How comprehend that the Second Amendment was to him as sacred as the First to me? This is the central divide of our nation, here in my living room. This is red-state-blue-state sundering blood and blood. Once when I described a pistol as "a weapon meant to kill a person," Tim objected with some heat, and I revised the sentence, "a weapon that could kill a person." But it felt inauthentic. There are at base two reasons for a gun: food and murder. What is the purpose of a pistol? Could I believe some myth of a passion for target practice? Could he?

He saved his spare hours for target practice. He took out a "lifetime subscription" to the NRA. He accreted knowledge, accuracy, skill. He learned how to dismantle and perfect a hammer, seer, and clip well. He invented an improved rifle sight. He acquired the ability to "checker" a grip with several hundred hair's-width grooves. He taught himself leatherwork—burning, carving, and lacing ammo belts and holsters. As I could walk into a fabric store, pass my hand over a bolt and tell you whether it was silk or fake, he could wander through a gun show and pick out a Norinco from a Chinese clone. As my father could rebuild a Plymouth, he could rebuild a Para-Ordnance P-14. As Peter knew basketball stats, Tim knew the specs of the Ruger and the Mauser.

I admired the concentration, the knowledge, the energy. I was proud of the dexterity, the perfectionist absorption. I was relieved by his rigorous attention to the permits and the safety rules.

Then he'd set a Walther PPK in my hand, and I was *embarrassed.*

———

Looking back through the trove of his letters, I found ample evidence that he "liked the risk"—of guns, the hunt, the jump. When he was in Airborne school he described the fall from an airplane with an adrenaline-soaked ardor that I had to believe sincere. "The plane is a rattletrap. The noise shakes

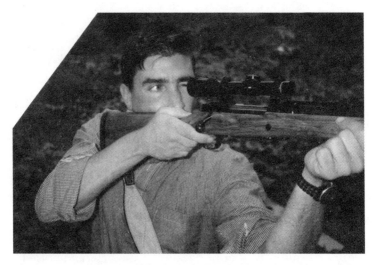

Almost any trip home to Tallahassee in the '80s and '90s.

you to the bone. And you come to the end of the rope, literally, and you know there's no way out but out that door. And you get to the door, it's your turn, and you go! And the silence you fall into is deeper than anything you ever dreamed."

Later he wrote a fictionalized, third-person account of a close call, a jump off course into trees when he felt "the rush of the slipstream," "the sudden gentle tug of his parachute," and the rote remembrance of his training:

> "... *don't release your ruck, keep your feet together but relaxed, so if you do hit the ground you can execute a dynamite PLF; last, just before you go beneath the first branch, tuck your chin on your chest and cover your face with your arms. When he had done all that—it took only a second to remember it and do it—he had only just enough time to wonder if he was going to get hurt before the black shadow of the trees darkened the air around*

him. His parachute caught in the top of a pine tree and the top of an oak, the two trees acting as a brake. His downward momentum was stopped, except for the stretch in the nylon cord that connected him to the circle of silk above his head. The suspension lines had just enough stretch to allow his feet to kiss the forest floor."

In these years, and especially later in Namibia, his attitude toward hunting veered in the direction of the mystical.

"I can't express how magical it was to be out in the veld again. The cold crisp air chilling you as you wait for shooting light. Watching the sunsets that you only find in Namibia. Sitting by the fire and remembering the day over a well earned dop with a best friend. The smell of a camelthorn fire. The sudden shortness of breath, as a slight movement turns into the ear of a graceful kudu or hardy gemsbok. The exhilaration of seeing a well-placed shot do its work. The sadness of a beautiful animal on the ground…"

The hunt involved him in rituals of kinship and gratitude to the animal:

"…I put my hand on the buck's head and wished him well, many ewes and green grass. I took a blade of grass and wet it in my mouth and then put it in his. I thanked him for his life, his hide, meat and horns, and the memory he has given me… Pieter called me over to the back of the bakkie and sliced open the heart… he blooded me, saying that this was the blood from the heart of my first gemsbok and would ensure that I never forgot this buck…"

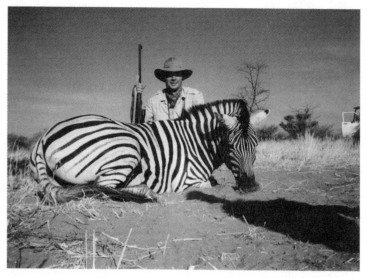

Namibian kill, c. 2000

This was still more alien to me, manly to the point of pompous, though I knew that the ceremonies derived from Africa and native America and had for Tim the force of religious rite. When he hunted in Florida—that preserve of bubba and the baseball cap—he still honored the enterprise with an ascot and his wide-brimmed, rakish, wool felt Australian hunting hat.

We found this funny.

He was buried in that hat.

———

"If you're ever going to visit me in Africa, Mom, this is the place."

When Peter and I touched down in Windhoek in July of 1998, met by Tim *insouciant* in many-pocketed cargo shorts, it seemed to me that at thirty-four he'd come into his own.

More: that he'd found a home. He loved the muted taupes and lavenders of the Namibian hills, the flaring sunsets, the vast distances cut through by a black wire of two-lane highway. He loved the sudden apparition of gamboling springbok, or the raw hunger of the hyenas prowling in ravines beside these roads. He loved the food, a legacy of German cuisine with a plethora of game. ("Chicken is considered a vegetable here.") He took to the off-hand conviviality of the veranda and the *braai*. He relaxed into a professional middle class where hunting was taken for granted as a sport. "Africa lite," he said.

And he was proud of the job, removing from the Angolan/Namibian border mines left there by the war between South Africa and SWAPO. He explained (heavy emphasis for Mom's sake on the safety of the method) how bulletproof bulldozers pushed the earth into furrows or "berms," in which the mines were then exploded by remote control.

He introduced us around the embassy and installed us in the "quarters" provided by the Army, a sprawling four-bedroom house with a wet bar, a pool, and a housekeeper's cottage (but the walls bare, the pool empty—another luxury barracks, a guy-house). Over beer while I slept, Tim admitted to Peter that he'd met a woman. He was reluctant to tell me because he assumed I'd consider it a betrayal of Jewel. Peter said he thought I would be relieved.

And I was relieved. Tim and Jewel had by now been eight years stuck in their ambivalent bond. Peter and I had been together for the same years and married for five of them, which I considered irresolution enough. I thought there came a point of impasse beyond which, if you could neither commit nor let go, mutual destruction lay.

So just as Namibia seemed a new start, Birgitt Coetzee seemed a new start. He brought her to meet us. Just half

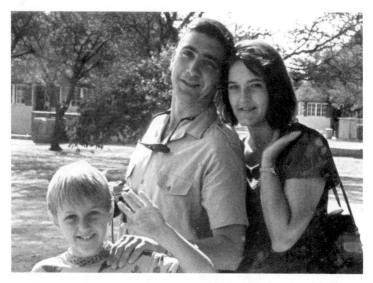

Neal, Tim and Birgitt on Safari, Namibia, 1998.

an hour at first, small talk and canapés. Birgitt was slender, pretty, articulate, energetic, and opinionated, with a confidence of carriage that may belong to Africa or may contrarily have signaled colonial entitlement. She was an information officer of the United Nations for Namibia—an impressive title concealing the fact, she explained, that she "did the work of an ex-pat on a local wage." She had an eight-year-old boy but no marriage in her past; this was an independent choice. She too had been raised by a single mother—who disliked Americans, but was "coming 'round"—Birgitt tilted her head flirtatiously at Tim—under the onslaught of his charm.

"Isn't her accent gorgeous?" When she'd gone Tim seemed nervous that we should like her, and I considered that a happy sign (at what point does a sixties mother begin to seek the stability for her children that she rejected for herself?). We'd liked her at once. Yes, her accent was delightful. We'd be glad to see more of her.

That first weekend Tim took Peter and me to Etjo Lodge on a private game preserve, where we ate gemsbok and kudu while black-and-white porcupines with a quill-span of three feet waddled begging across the kitchen. The next weekend we traveled in Tim's bakkie north to Etosha National Park with Birgitt and platinum-blond Neal. We stayed in simple government-run lodges, and Neal would slip in before dawn to jiggle Peter on the shoulder. "Peter! Peter! Get up! The elephants are at the water hole!"

Night in the lion blind: the King and one of his pride are thrown a haunch of springbok for their supper. Morning: twenty elephants and a dozen wildebeest congregate at the water's edge. More zebras than you can count. Ostrich. Ostrich. Hippo. Hippo. A lioness in the undergrowth. An angry rhinoceros. Termite skyscrapers. Giraffes calmly munching the upper leaves. Springbok in the culvert. Hyenas in the valley. More flamingos than you can count. Just this one more turnoff. Get the camera. Lion in the open. Yes. Back this way. Gemsbok. Kudu. Dik-dik. Zebra. More springbok than you can count.

Tim drove the bakkie with one hand on the wheel, cool. It reminded me of the guys in high school in the fifties with their necker-knobs. It reminded me of my dad, showing Yellowstone to Stan and me while we sulked in the backseat: *Just up this road. Just one more turnoff. There might be more mud bubbles over that hill just there. It might be the biggest geyser we've ever seen!*

When in 1999 Tim was cut loose from the Namibian embassy with the promise that he would be rehired as a civilian, it did not occur to me to ask what it portended, that the Army was demilitarizing one task in Africa. And indeed it would be three full years after Tim's suicide before the *New York Times* acknowledged civilian employees as a "shadow force in Iraq almost as large as the uniformed military," and five before we learned that the CIA had hired Blackwater to assassinate al-Qaeda operatives.

In the meantime, while Tim waited for clearance he moved back into his Tallahassee apartment (makeshift furniture, bullet-filling machine) and went to work as a "technical recruiter," which meant a headhunter of computer geeks. The work was dreary, self-thwarting, and more deadening than finance.

And I did sometimes think the situation made *his head go all wonky*. One day at work Tim was at the Xerox machine while a woman co-worker picked up trash. The company vice president came in and said to the woman, "Give me your arm." He took hold of it and used it to slap Tim across the face, hard enough to leave a welt. Then the VP laughed and said, "I didn't hit you! She did!"

There was apparently no intention behind this crassness but a crass joke. But Tim was incensed, outraged. He tried cooling off for a weekend but did not cool off. He wrote the Veep's boss calling the incident "harassment" and "battery." He filed a police report.

His reaction was of a piece with his rigorous law-abiding code. But I thought it, and Peter thought it, over the top. *Let it go*, we urged him. *The guy's an ass. It's not worth the loss of sleep.*

Later, in similar outrage in Namibia, Tim sued a bank that had repossessed his "bakkie," a jeep-like truck for which he had paid cash—had paid it, as it turned out, to a criminal well known to the bank. In this instance he was clearly in the right, but in both it disturbed me that my own off-spring seemed to be buying into the American zest for a legal battle—all those boiling cups of coffee, cockroaches in the hotdogs, nieces who thought they should be compensated for the terror of their uncles as the plane went down.

I think it must have been during the fight with the Veep in Tallahassee, when Tim was spending weekends reading guy-trash novels beside the pool, that he said, "If it wasn't for what it would do to you, I'd kill myself." I say *I think it must have been*, and this bemuses and amazes me, that I could have heard this sentence and not memorized the date and hour. I now think his anger and obsession were a displacement of a conflict within, and that what did not seem dangerous because it was irrational was in fact a signal of danger because it was irrational.

Peter advised him to rejoin the Army. The drawdown was over and they were looking for officers again. "You were happiest there," Peter urged. I did not then know that his superior officers in Stuttgart had recommended him for "return to active duty now. Promote immediately to major…Top pick for line Battalion Command." To re-enlist would mean giving up Birgitt, Namibia, and family life. It doesn't surprise me that he didn't lay this option before me. He would have known that if he decided on that military path I would accept it, but he wouldn't have wanted to hear my advice. Nor did I ask him how and when he had disentangled himself from his long relationship with Jewel. I assumed that he would be honest with her. I didn't want to pry.

In the event, after six months the necessary clearances came through, and Tim stored his goods and hugged us good-bye at the familiar airport barrier.

———

A year and a half later: "You should come to the wedding, Mom. I'm only going to do this once," he said.

But it was fourteen hours by plane from England. We had two weeks off from teaching, and London for Christmas was already a major effort in so short a time. Classes would begin the first week of January. There'd be jet lag. Classes to prepare. Every headline predicted disaster at Y2K: computers would go haywire, worldwide air traffic control would break down. Africa wasn't the best place to be aloft in an apocalypse.

I told Tim, "I don't think we'd die. I just think I'd be so nervous it would spoil the occasion."

Instead we flew home. It was easy to get tickets—nobody wanted to travel on New Year's Eve. And we'd be back before midnight in case the world came to a standstill.

We were over the Atlantic when they married, Birgitt in zebra-patterned chiffon and Tim in the tux I'd sent from London, on the top of a hill with a view of the setting sun that was still riding cloud-tops where we sat in our Delta socks.

We were home by seven. Watched the chaos at Trafalgar Square on the tube and went to bed, figuring to be up at midnight to greet the millennium EST. But slept right through.

11.

Houston, May 2005. Gary Pitts turned out to be a tall, unaffected, and slightly gangly blond, while opposing counsel Roger Levy affected a slicked-back shiny-suited shyster mode, enjoying himself by way of sarcasm and theatrical exasperation. We gathered in the courthouse where a scant year later the Enron scandal would unfold. There was a scheduling glitch, so we cooled our heels in the waiting room through the morning and the afternoon, Gary busily re-ordering the massive stack of exhibits Birgitt had gathered, me performing squats to limber up my spine, Peter urging calm, Birgitt keeping up her energy with little bursts of impatience.

Birgitt's German-Namibian psychiatrist had been deposed, testifying that Tim had suffered from PTSD. But for all the symptoms Tim had shown—hypervigilance, hyper-arousal, irritability, fear, depression—no one could say for sure that he had "reliving" flashbacks, and this by Dr. Sieber-hagen's admission was a problem for "making the diagnosis in the technically correct manner." At some point during the morning Gary brought in an affidavit from the opposing counsels' psychiatric witness, which we read passing each page from hand to hand. This "expert" went meticulously through all the same information as Birgitt's and came to directly opposite conclusions. No sign of PTSD. Tim's suicide was the result of domestic conflict.

Peter and I could not then foresee that Birgitt's case would lurch through six years of judgment, review, mediation, and appeal while she pressed doggedly on, nor that the DBA insurance companies' success in denying benefits would eventually land them in congressional investigation. But we did at that moment understand that the outcome came down to a *he said/he said* between two psychiatrists neither of whom had seen Tim in his lifetime, and that such an exchange was unlikely to end in unequivocal triumph.

We were called to the courtroom late in the afternoon, and through the evening and the next day the lawyers circled through Tim's life, his time in Iraq, and his last weeks, energetically seeking to prove some point that seemed to me peripheral. I was here voluntarily. I wanted Birgitt to win her suit. But it was not my fight, and somehow not emotionally within my grasp.

Gary strove to prove Tim lived at an impairing pitch of stress. Levy characterized Tim's job as "office management," denigrating Tim as just the kind of apparatchik he went to Iraq to avoid being. Birgitt grew tired, and fatigue made her answers brittle.

At noon of the second day she went to pack for her return flight, and I took the stand. The court reporter had me raise my right hand—there was no bible—and said, "Do you solemnly swear that the testimony you are about to give is the truth?" No *whole truth*, no *nothing but the truth*—and my brain dawdled among these interesting omissions. I wondered whether the law had by now acknowledged that there is no possible way of telling the whole truth. Once in a textbook I wrote that there is a curious prejudice built into our language that makes us speak of "telling *a* lie" but "telling *the* truth," as if lies were multiple and various but truth were a single whole. "*Telling a lie* is a truer phrase than *telling the truth*," I'd written. Now it occurred to me that any "whole truth" must take in impressions, guesses, intuition—all the things that are inadmissible in a court of law and that are yet forms of knowledge on which we base our best notion of what truth might be if it were whole. I wondered if the law had come to recognize that swearing on the Christian bible was not a universal guarantee of veracity, which would signal—wouldn't it?—the narrowing of the globe, acknowledgement of the Muslim world, not to mention the Jewish, Hindu, Buddhist—perhaps even the agnostic worlds? All this was playing in my head before I had been asked a question.

Gary asked for a summary of Tim's life, which I narrated—jobs, countries, companies. He asked about the Ethiopian Project Tim had previously headed up for RONCO. No, I said, Tim didn't tell me that one of his men had lost a foot to a mine explosion. Yes, I did know that the whole family had suffered from illness there—giardia, rotavirus, malaria. Gary asked about Tim's character, and I said that, though his military interest was foreign to me, "You know, he was the kind—he was the unusual kind of boy who, if you said *take out the garbage*—he took out the garbage. My younger son was a totally different sort."

The judge interjected that he'd had the different sort.

My voice may have been a little rough through this recital. When we took a break the judge came down to the witness box, asked if I was all right, and called for someone to bring me water. But in fact I felt no distress, only that I was something of an automaton until his kindness momentarily threatened to break through to me. Perhaps the courtroom seemed unreal because the magnitude of things was reversed, the large business of death and justice reduced to these talking suits and pieces of paper in a stack, whereas the mundane reality of a life—"Hiya, Mom," "Hello the house!"—had been flung out into the unanswerable vast.

———

The trial left Peter swollen with contained anger that Tim had been subjected to this bandying of his motives and circumstances. For me he was simply absent from a proceeding that had the power neither to deny nor confer his "honor." It took me several months to realize that what the court *had* conferred—stripped of the personalities, the trappings of courtroom drama, my own benumbed performance anxiety—were hundreds of pages of clues to what Tim's life had been like through his ordeal in Iraq. I began to comb through emails and "exhibits."

I learned two things at once: that the danger had risen sharply through his weeks in Iraq, and that he could be recognizably himself and still present a different self to each audience. In emails to me he was devil-may-care, confiding but always with a hint of swagger; to stepmother Barbi bluff and practical; with Birgitt more open about danger, incompetence, and injustice; with his friends jokey and sometimes testy; in his RONCO reports at first steadily optimistic, and then more urgent, and finally demanding or angrily sounding the alarm.

In his first news of the Iraq assignment he assured me that he and his men would be operating "almost exclusively 'inside the wire,' which means that we are surrounded by all kinds of military units with lots of firepower"—as if that would reassure me. But I replied in kind, "With a tiny bit of heart-in-throat, I'm proud o' ya." He finished the Ethiopian project with only a few days to wind down in Namibia before he flew off to Kuwait, and touched down in Baghdad a week later

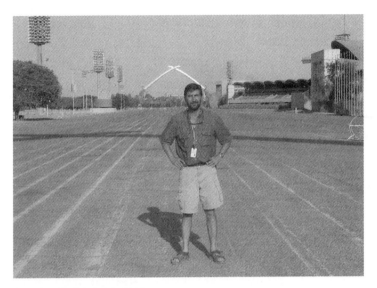

Arrival in Baghdad, July 2003.

in temperature of 52 Celsius. He complained, in that familiar proud-grousing tone, that he and his skeleton team were unsatisfactorily bunked in "Saddam's major palace in an open bay with two or three hundred other folks."

Through September his team was refurbishing its training quarters not far from the palace, beside the 14th of July Bridge. I demanded a map of Baghdad sufficiently detailed that I could X his spot. By early October he was "pretty impressed with my Iraqis so far." He claimed that safety was no problem, because "we spend the majority of our time in a golden prison of the U.S. secure area." He boasted a collection of military rifles and machine guns and was looking forward to the next Thursday, "when we go and look at a 20 foot container of weapons at one of the collection points for the Coalition." That weekend on the phone to Peter he exulted that he'd "scored an AK-47."

On October 26 there was a rocket attack on the hotel Al-Rasheed that killed an American colonel, and sent Secretary Paul Wolfowitz scurrying for safety. Tim dashed out an email: "We are all fine and not involved..." I replied more or less flippantly, "I feel embarrassed that I am not more worried about you...I am participating in your toughness the only way I can. Love you. Do you want cookies?"

But the next day one of the palaces and the Red Cross were hit, and I recanted. "I take it back. Today's four bombs seemed aimed at precisely the sort of operation you run..." Tim replied with the usual bravado. "We are well screened by other civilian buildings and we are not a target worth spending resources [on]."

———

Kids lie to their parents. I knew this. I had suffered my own lies as the major grief of my adolescence, and as a consequence had made it the touchstone of my parenting: my boys would be able to tell me *anything*. Did I think my need for openness automatically dovetailed with *their* needs? How many lies had I told my mother and father as my marriage foundered, because it was easier on me to be easier on them? But sitting at my computer looking out my Florida window while my son sat sweating at his computer in Iraq, it suited me to think he was pursuing his adventure, just as it suited him to let me think so.

Painfully now, two years later at the same desk, I encountered the coda to his letter:

"Funny about age. Coming up on 40, I realize that I'm not 20-something any more, and don't feel old at all. Remember being 20 and thinking that 40 was ancient

and on the slippery slope to death. Now realizing we're only halfway done."

That was October. He was only halfway done with Iraq. The same day, he wrote to a colleague that the situation was "sobering," and in his weekly report to RONCO that the security situation was "significantly more dangerous." They had established safe rooms at their quarters. He worried about his men out in the field "being caught in crossfire."

In November there was another mortar attack near the palace inside the Green Zone, in Fallujah two American civilians were killed, and at the demolition site shots were fired at his men. Twice on the phone with Tim, Birgitt heard bombs nearby. She admitted to watching the news "perversely relieved when it says soldier and not contractor..." To the Washington office Tim wrote worrying that the team's insurance "was not effective if death or injury was a result of 'acts of war.' Could you please check it out for all of us here in Iraq?" In December his men were fired on again, and operations were suspended. Some of the Iraqi workers were threatened with death unless they stopped working with the Americans. One left Baghdad and another resigned.

Tim began to warn of significant morale problems, there being "no places to safely go." He argued forcefully, a little angrily, for more frequent R&R, faster rotation of his expat men. To a friend on the RONCO staff he wrote,

"Let's see, first I put on my pistol then my body armor... then my equipment vest. Double check I have four IDs and do a check of my cell phone, sat phone and VHF radio and lastly do I have my smoke grenades, charge my MP5... check my G3 and the extra

mags for all of the above. Are we doing Humanitarian Demining?"

"How are you?" I asked as a matter of course, again, another-gain at the beginning of every phone call. "Survivin', survivin'." I always took this to mean: *okay, not great.* I sometimes heard it as a prelude to a rant I didn't want to hear, about this one's failure of honesty, that one's greed. Now I wondered how often, its opposite implied, this was the literal news: *I am surviving.*

In his January monthly report, the last I have, Tim recorded, "Attacks against civilian/contractors continue and are a major concern. In addition...the threat of kidnapping has now arisen." Scrawled sloppily, unpunctuated, across his daily planner among schoolboy doodles of missiles, bombs, rifles, and hand grenades, he wrote:

all mistakes anyway everything crazy now I hope I can make it home safe.

Gary had said Birgitt's case could prevail by showing that Tim's "exposure to the 'special zone of danger' in Iraq aggravated or accelerated his preexisting psychic condition." But this was not the case. *Preexisting condition* is insurance-speak for *claim denied.* The French in World War I refused to recognize the phenomenon of shell shock by blaming "preexisting conditions" for all subsequent mental breakdown. An estimate by British authorities puts at over three hundred, in the same war, the number of soldier shell-shock victims executed for cowardice. In the First Gulf War, V.A. doctors recognized as a distinct group those "most genetically vulnerable" to Sarin nerve gas, but not to PTSD or suicide. In Iraq, American soldiers suffering from clinical depression and post-traumatic stress were treated with drugs and sent back into combat.

Everyone has a preexisting condition. Everyone has DNA, a childhood, a temperament, a circumstance, a history, baggage. You go to war with the wounds you have. I was reminded of a lawyer friend in Belgium forty years ago (Tim would have been just toddling, chubby-legged, gossamer-haired, methodically making his way from Bauhaus coffee table to bent-tube chair) who pointed out that the law is at least as much concerned with order as with truth and justice. "Take the side of the road," he suggested. "There's no morality attaching to the left or right. It's a question of the law imposing order, and *after that* it becomes immoral to drive on the other side." In Tim's case the law seemed to dictate that *irresistible impulse* was on one side of the road, meaning benefits for his wife and children, and *suicidally depressed* was on the other, meaning none.

———

The post-trial depositions were passed along by Gary's office, and I read over again the words of people I had never met before Tim died, who saw the affable friend, and saw him change: "...it came in spurts. Some days he was completely normal, like his old self. And then sometimes you would see this—you would see that he did not react, that he was somewhere else with his thoughts."

Among these pages I came across a passage of cross-examination about why Tim had said, "I'm tired of being the bad man." For Birgitt it was just weirdly unlike Tim. "There is no context to it. I can't explain it. It was things he said just out of the blue..." She remembered that twice, in the car, he had turned up the radio to hear a song that "says something with a bad man and behind blue eyes and biting back on your anger." But this made no sense to her. "Bad about what? He wasn't bad."

I Googled "bad man behind blue eyes" and there popped up on the screen the lyrics of the song that I vaguely remembered from the seventies:

> *"No one knows what it's like*
> *To be the bad man*
> *To be the sad man*
> *Behind blue eyes . . .*

It spoke so clearly of the self-concealment of depression that it was as if I was tossed back into the years post-divorce:

> *"But my dreams*
> *They aren't as empty*
> *As my conscience seems to be . . .*

I went to the mall and found a cover by Limp Bizkit that the clerk said had been played on the radio worldwide in 2003:

> *"No one knows what it's like*
> *to feel these feelings*
> *like I do, and I blame you!*
> *No one bites back as hard*
> *on their anger . . ."*

I showed the lyrics to Julia Kling. She said, "Oh. It's his note."

I thought: *his tone, his sound?* "His note?"

"His suicide note, I mean."

A memory—"*there is no context to it*"—surfaces. Toward the end of our eight-month stay in Illinois, Tim had two molars pulled at a local dental clinic. I was at the nadir of depression then, had been teaching with such dread that I arrived at class fifteen minutes early just so I could hold onto the steering wheel and deep-breathe before going to the classroom. We'd all had indifferent dental care in England, and I was nursing a dull toothache myself, but Tim's mouth-mess was dire. I delivered him into the hands of the white-uniformed assistant and sat with a tattered magazine in my lap. I can see the text dancing in front of me, my imagination at work on the fear and loathing of my eight-year-old inside: the smell of the gas, the taste of blood, the whirring of instruments like metal insects. I'm pretty hard-nosed about hospitals, but then, there, I was sick with the mother-knowledge that I could do nothing for him. The minutes went by in countable seconds. I doubted once again that I could go through with this, launching out on my own with two dependent lives attached to me by two-ton cable. I was called into the recovery room where, mouth spilling gauze as if he had been gagged, blood bubbling from his nose, Tim emerged with painful slowness into consciousness. I thought: *I can't do this. What made me think I could do this? The boys will be better off with their father. I can't cope.*

I'm not a psychologist, though I have been guided by two of the best in life and many more in literature, and for forty years it has been a pleasure to explore with Julia Kling the myriad ways writing fiction is like psychological practice. "Practice" may be the operative word. My reading of Tim's life inevitably works by analogy, both because that is how a fiction writer thinks and because I am conscious of traits I had in common with my son. Samuel Johnson describes how, in the method of biography, joy and sorrow for someone else's life is produced by an act of imagination "that realizes the event, however fictitious, or approximates it, however remote, by placing us, for a time, in the condition of him whose fortune we contemplate."

Restlessly since Tim's death I have tried to place myself in the condition (however fictitious, however remote) of him whose fortune I contemplate. So I count backwards through Tim's forebears looking for a clue to his character: The great-great-grandfather who joined the Union Army and later drank; his wife who turned him out; the great-grandmother who defied the Germans; the Scottish prohibitionist; the grand-uncle who wrote nutty "Infiniverse;" the Taft Republican banker; the Bauhaus architect who killed himself; the historian academic; the daredevil pilot; the news editor on the *L.A. Times*; the architect for Euratom. I watch this march of ancestors and can see offered forth for Tim's chromosomes, art, alcohol, the love of risk, meticulousness, and moralism. There are, I also see, those who died too early and those who lived beyond expectation.

I am told that Tim's father, in his later years, when he was on the bipolar downswing would take a bottle into a room and immure himself for days. I had roller-coaster moods myself in my younger years, though a doctor explained to me that I was not a "manic-depressive" because (like Tim) I could function in both high and low states. It's also true that when I gave up alcohol my moods evened out. In any case, it's likely that a chemical imbalance was something that Tim inherited from both his parents. For Walter, the multiple crises of the theatre kept depression at bay. Tim, needing extreme stimulus to keep himself charged with adrenaline, found the Army for that high, and when he tried to modulate toward a normal life could not stop the descent into the depression he became adept at hiding.

In many ways I shared Tim's perfectionism, overintensity, arrogance. We had in common a love of company, an extreme need for solitude, and difficulty balancing these incompatible desires. We both loved feeling competent and watching competence in others. We were alike driven to be productive and intolerant of being told what to do.

But, for all its melodrama, my life has led toward reconciliation. There is not the contradiction between mothering and literature that there is between fathering and war. The central conflict of my life, the need for family and the need to write, has led me a merry chase through compromise—typing with a baby on my lap, settling hour by hour for the lesser pleasures of the classroom, putting off the chapter for the homework or the macaroni or the Little League.

Here's the irony: that nothing led me toward eventual adulthood quite so insistently as the passive endurance of my disappointment—that I had borne, and must adore, a golden right-wing gun-toting soldier son.

"As troops begin to rotate out of Iraq and Afghanistan, they are being met by communities that often have no concept of how to help reintegrate them into society." So says Stephen L. Robinson of the National Gulf War Resource Center, in an assessment written for the progressive think tank Center for American Progress in 2004. To a certain extent this is true in any war. You can read it in the novels and memoirs of the two World Wars. The family circle closes because its members are forced to function without the father. Once he returns there is strain as the hoop is pulled apart to fit him

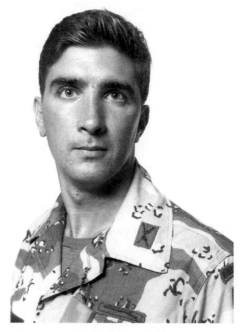

Soldier son, c. 1989.

in again. For the returning soldier or contractor, having been immersed in a situation of intensity and vigilance leads him to find domestic life banal, trivial, enervating.

Birgitt is the first to say that she was ignorant of depression and unresponsive to Tim's struggle. "It never dawned on me that he was deadly serious...that something was seriously amiss," she said. "I thought you had to have a reason to be depressed, and he had no reason."

But nobody knows what it's like to be the bad man. In the public mind, the word "contractor" applies equally to the corporations that obtain the government contract and the employees such company hires to do the work. Both are equally tainted with the greed and carelessness of human life that Tim saw at RONCO. Namibia, too, is in some ways a special case. I think Tim's friends were completely supportive of him personally, but this was a former German colony with an ancient undercoat of anti-Americanism, and feeling against the war in Iraq was nearly universal. Younger, savvier citizens ridiculed the posturing-monkey U.S. President. Ilke had put on the refrigerator a cartoon of Saddam with his mouth open for inspection, the doctor asking, "Any WMD's in there? At Christmas Tim found this funny. In April he coldly turned on his heel.

Over and over again in the literature of war's aftermath—Iraq in this respect no different from any other—you read of the warrior's longing for a normal life, the "honeymoon" period when he is back home again, then the shift. Scott Anderson, writing in the *New York Times Magazine*, describes it, "For some it was simple boredom, while others described it as a restlessness they couldn't shake...[or] it was worse...like being trapped in an elevator that won't stop dropping." Anderson notes something else working away at demobilized men: "the often utterly irrational guilt that took hold of them when something went wrong."

————

It's most often late at night that I come face to face with Tim's last days, knowing that *no one knows what it was like* for him, but asking what it was like, making it up, imagining the conversation we will never have. Every parent of a dead child I have known talks to him, to her. It isn't necessary to believe in ghosts.

A strange thing I continue to learn is that it doesn't hurt to talk *about* him. A cup of coffee, a phone call, dinner, the Internet—among friends I am eager to connect with them, not Tim. Speaking objectifies him and so sets his loss at a remove. And when I'm writing I have verbal nails and miters, planes and levels, a shed's worth of cared-for tools to give me the illusion of control.

Once when I was six, visiting my grandparents in Wilcox on my own, Gamie gave me a stack of old Christmas cards to play with, and as I looked up from them through the window into the yard—the weeping willow, the washtub, Weedy the Pekinese chasing a pie pan—I was whacked in the stomach with an incorporeal pain. Gamie saw my face. "Why, what's the matter?" I said, "I don't *know*," and she said, "Oh, dolly, you're homesick." I made her spell it. I wrote a letter: "I am *homesick*." It was the first time I understood this transformative consolation: if there was a word for it, I was not alone. If there was a word, it had been in the world before. The link from that moment to these pages is absolute.

I am homesick for you, Tim.

So last thing before I fall asleep I press my hand against my clavicle where I supported your newborn head—there is nothing of you there now but the moisture on my palm—and go over what I can know of what it was like behind your blue eyes.

I see you in the open bakkie in twilight, with Pieter and two or three of his staff, the truck juddering over the rough ground past stands of kokerboom and thorn and mopane trees, past springbok and little dik-dik, you not happy because you don't like to cull, would rather hunt on foot at dawn. You aim awkwardly because your own rifle is not zeroed and this is one of Pieter's guns. You hit a gemsbok, see it stagger and bound among the trees, and jump down to follow, but now it grows too dark for tracking. Next morning you are up in half-light, but another herd has already covered up the spoor. You find a tooth and know you shot the animal in the face. I don't know whether you must punish yourself by putting a gun to your face, but I think it possible. What I feel sure of is that, having left the animal to die, you experience it as the abandoning of your men. I do not think this is fanciful on my part, even if it was on yours. Alvarez says, "The world of the suicide is superstitious, full of omens…he enters a shut-off, impregnable world where everything fits." I experienced this myself when I was just your age, believing coincidences were cosmic messages. Now I think of the ceramic horse given you by your Iraqi men, its leg broken in transit (in that mammoth suitcase I sent for your birthday, wrapped in your dirty T-shirts?), which you could not repair, and which *you* made clear was a symbol of breaking faith with them.

I can only guess what happens the next night, the last night, at the reserve. But I think that of all people Pieter, best man, best friend, is the one to whom you would lay out your dilemma: you made a deal with Birgitt that you'd do two years in Washington. You can't expect her to be satisfied playing *hausfrau*. But now that debt is due, you can't face a sedentary job in the very place you see as the source of blundering and lies. You're back in the same spot you were with Jewel, having to stay stateside for the sake of her career. But leaving the marriage is not an option: *I'm only going to do this once.* I think Pieter says: *If that's the case, you must take your stand with Birgitt.* He'd say some way or other: *Be a man.* This is me making fiction. I know nothing of what happened. But it would explain why Pieter would not come to the funeral, would send no message but, "I can't think of Tim that way."

I see you back at home, not having slept, banging the binoculars against the table, saying you will take them back to the store where the gunsmith sold away the gun you ordered.

"My God, I hate dishonest people." You tell Birgitt you're depressed, not just about the wounded buck, but about the rifle, the bakkie court case, your guys in Iraq.

No one is overwhelmed by one thing. When depression descends, the smallest of mundane tasks—brushing your teeth, putting on your shoes—becomes a daunting burden. Then there is a minute solace in the exercise of will, a limiting of focus that temporarily blocks the dark. Two things men use to displace despair: anger and errands. So you rouse yourself, marching with military vigor through the house. You cross-check figures on your mother-in-law's estate, go to the hardware store, mail RONCO shirts to Iraq, compile and deliver a set of GPS maps to Pieter's house, pick up Neal and Thyra, try to put Thyra down for a nap.

And do you at that point go for a drink, out of Birgitt's sight? So easy to do, as I know from my own long experience.

And if at that point the phone should ring? If, hemispheres away, both north and west, I should be on the line? *How are you?* and you would say, *Survivin', survivin'*—and would I hear by how thin a thread that is so? and would I know how to save you, as my much-maligned mother saved me once, in some adolescent grief, when I picked up the phone in the dorm basement and called collect: *Mom, I'm in trouble,* and she said, *Come home.* But I was half your age, and a girl, and could admit to trouble. I had not built, was not responsible for, an edifice of new lives and old ideals.

In any case there is no such call. You try to put Thyra down for a nap. She senses your brusqueness, even your unhappiness. She, unusually, screams for her mother. You slam the door. Neal too defies you, and Birgitt intervenes. How can they know from how long ago and how heavily the cascade falls? They never signed up for the warrior's dream.

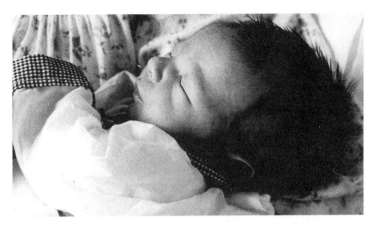

One day old; Feb. 25, 1964.

I think you bite back the angry thing you want to shout, as the father shouted who "taught you how not to be a father." The flood of failures rises: the hunter, the gunsmith, the litigant, the patriot, the American, the soldier, the entrepreneur, the husband, the father. All ineffectual, all shot to shit. You're tired of being the bad man. No one knows what it's like. To feel these feelings. To be telling only lies. Empty conscience, love as vengeance, never free.

———

I don't know whether any of this is as I say. I don't know, if you had lived on, how much you might have changed, or whether "Get me some help" was an accusation or a plea. I don't know whether it was your settled intent to pull the trigger, or whether, having done so, you had a split second for regret. Alvarez says he believes there is "a whole class of suicides...who take their own lives not in order to die but to escape confusion, to clear their heads." For such persons suicide operates as an "unencumbered reality" that allows them to "break through the patterns of obsession and necessity which they have unwittingly imposed upon their lives."

I don't know whether this is relevant. The point of the exercise seems to be to teach myself that I don't know, that when all is said and done, which must of necessity be said and done, the task of grief is to accept that the only blue eyes I can see behind are my own.

I press my palm against my collarbone, stroking the crown of your newborn head. "It's all right," I say. "It'll be all right."

I don't know what I mean.

12.

I remember an evening, perhaps in 1992. Tim was back from Hawaii and in love with Jewel. Peter and I were together but not yet married. The four of us had eaten dinner at Peter's house and sat with coffee afterward, Peter leaning back in his chair with the ease that means *laid back*. Tim was clean-shaven and Army-shorn. Jewel's hair fell luxurious to mid-arm, that color called "raven" not because it is black but because it has the iridescent sheen of feathers. There may have been some talk of prospective marriage, either theirs or ours, because Peter said smiling, "I think ordinary daily life is vastly underrated."

Jewel grinned. Tim gave a little shake of his head.

I laughed. "Oh, yes. The real adventure is in the living room." This time Tim's headshake was deliberate and emphatic. "No way," he said.

How many times did he tell me—warn me—that he was ready to die for his country, rushing full tilt and willing into battle? How can it have come about that he died violently at home?

I asked John McBride, who was closest to him since fifth grade, if he had a theory. John said at once, "Unenlightened chivalry."

———

In the years since the invasion of Iraq, there has been a general gingerliness around the issue of "supporting our troops," a nationwide pussy-footing that has gained no purchase with the length and cost of two ill-considered wars. This note is typical, from a letter to the editor in *The New York Times*: "The discussion should not be about the nobility or honor of the young people who enlisted in the military to fight the 'war on terror.' There is no question about that..."

I want to question it.

I want to question it because there is no such discussion, and because this preemptive disclaimer represents a national cowardice. To "give support" to a widow or a cancer victim means to empathize with a state of loss or fear, whereas to "support the troops" means to cheer them uncritically on their mission. More: rhetorical voices are raised to reassert our democratic right to impugn the government, whereas we still fear as unpatriotic examining the motives of many thousands of teenagers with multifarious backgrounds, intelligence, proclivities, and rates of maturation who may or may not have understood what they were getting into. A combination of youthful exuberance, yearning, and testosterone makes young men especially vulnerable to a campaign of persuasion intrinsic to our politics, older than Thermopylae and as cool as MTV: *honor and nobility lie this way.*

Chris Hedges, in *War Is a Force That Gives Us Meaning*, tries to account for the temptation: "Many young men, schooled in the notion that war is the ultimate definition of manhood, that only in war will they be tested and proven, that they can discover their worth as human beings in battle, willingly join the great enterprise." For such young men "the high-blown rhetoric" and "the ideal of nobility beckon [them] forward."

If these young men are hoodwinked into a certain brand of order, sold on a promise of glory and nobility by the same means as they are hooked into Action Man, PlayStation, and Big Mac, we may not say so. It would undermine the troops. It would give aid and comfort to the enemy.

———

Another memory burbles up: the boys and I were in London together, which means it was 1975, which means they were and nine and eleven. Evel Knievel was scheduled to jump his motorcycle over thirteen London double-decker buses at Wembley Stadium. Tim was keen to go, and Alex had already been treated to Don McLean at the Royal Albert Hall, so (rolling my eyes even then, as I remember, at the oddity of pre-teen boys) I bought "good" tickets and we wended our way by tube and bus to where tens of thousands sat, and took our place on flat first-section benches where neither of them could really see. The Knievel stunt would take only a few minutes, and the impresarios had to give us our money's worth, so a minor fleet of emblazoned cycles zipped across the grounds on high wires for half an hour. Then the main warm-up act was announced, a dive from a hundred-foot platform into a bucket-deep wading pool by a fellow who was seventy-some years old. This wouldn't take long either, so we were treated to fifteen minutes of loudspeaker build-up about how dangerous it was, what could happen if the old fellow miscalculated by just an inch, what parts of his body could sustain such-and-such damage—on and on. The fellow did us a pantomime of terror up on the platform. The audience tired of the ballyhoo and began to slow-clap. The fellow dived. It was his thing; he was fine. The audience was not impressed.

I don't remember exactly how the Knievel stunt was set up then, the thirteen buses driven from left and right into place or some such show, while the barker used that amplified r-r-rolling basso that drums up avidity for circuses, basket-ball, and NASCAR: "Layyyy-dees and Gennnn-tlemennn…" Knievel appeared and mounted the motorcycle and adjusted this and that and this again. *Vroom-vroom.* Everybody stood. Tim and Alex, in unison with several thousand other child-spectators, climbed onto their seats. At last Knievel gunned it and took off up the wooden slope, flew into the mild evening air—and didn't make it. I think his back wheel caught against the roof of the thirteenth bus. I think he landed bone-break-ingly sideways, skidding on the down ramp and skewing off into the dirt. I didn't see it. I had, wimp mother, smashed my face into the stomach of eleven-year-old Tim, who excitedly comforted me—the oxymoron is accurate—"He'll be okay, Mom. He's done it before. He's really *brave!*"

———

There's a photographer named Tim Page who became famous for his wrenching shots of the killers and the dead of Vietnam. Years after the war had ended, he was asked by a publisher to choose a selection of his work that they would produce in an anthology "to take the glamour out of war once and for all." Page declined. He makes a "duh!" face to the TV camera and spreads his hands. "How can you do that? What could you find to thrill you? Might as well try to take the glamour out of sex."

Chris Hedges again: "War is necrophilia…hidden under platitudes about duty or comradeship.…When we spend long enough in war it comes to us as a kind of release, a fatal and seductive embrace that can consummate the long flirta-tion in war with our own destruction." The ancient Greeks, he says, described heroes with the word *ekpyrosis*, which means "to be consumed by a ball of fire."

———

"He was not dedicated to any silly crusade against land mines," Rob had said, which was true, although, thinking about the work Tim did over the years, I myself came to see the mines and their removal as a paradigm—I might say a cartoon—of mankind making the earth uninhabitable for mankind. Wars are fought over territory that mines make equally lethal for those who come to claim or reclaim, invade or build upon. The mine is a manufactured object with the express purpose of self-destructing and is hugely cost-effective. One can be bought for about the price of a Dove ice cream bar in an airport, but costs a thousand dollars to remove—which is one-third the price of a prosthetic limb.

———

I am thinking now of two insights into the "warrior spirit" or "unenlightened chivalry." One is Gary Pitts's notion, earned out of his own experience, that "[t]he military . . . fills a void in those who long for honor, loyalty, stability and sense of belonging." The other is from Thomas Joiner's *Why People Die by Suicide*, in which he posits that "successful" self-destruction occurs in those who have habituated themselves to hardship, pain, and danger. Suicide is not about weakness, he says, but requires "the fearless endurance of a certain type of pain." And this fearlessness, like any skill, requires practice. "People cannot develop the ability to lethally injure themselves quickly; the experiences that are required take time and repetition."

Joiner does not in any way glamorize the uniquely grim "courage or strength" that suicide requires. Nor does he deal at any length with the military's deliberate, daily, and repetitive habituation to pain and danger. But in the juxtaposition of these two insights is a possible answer to the high rates of suicide among war veterans. The young man who looks for honor and belonging finds it in the context of danger and daring. When exhilaration and adrenaline are left behind, the consciousness of honor and belonging also wither. It is hard, then, to deal with the pallid adventure of the living room.

———

A BBC documentary on the "band of brothers" plays with these ideas. There is an innate human desire for family, it says, such that a standard tactic used by military organizations (including street gangs, resistance fighters, terrorists, and suicide bombers) is to separate the young person from his original kin in favor of a substitute "fictive family." All successful ideological groups use the metaphor of family, which echoes among the *fathers* of the Catholic Church and the *brethren* of the Protestants, the *fraternities* and *sororities* of academia, the *sisterhood* of feminists, and the *brothahs* and *sistahs* of black power. It is inherent in *God the father, God the son.* The military in particular seeks out young people who can be brought to accept the substitute, which is then ritually idealized. Like families, the banded brothers are responsible for each other, loyal to each other, together beyond death. They play out these loyalties in situations that blazingly reinforce the sense of mutual dependency.

The idea is very old, pervasive, and persuasive. In *Luke*, Jesus is asked by a prospective disciple to please "suffer me first to go and bury my father," to which Jesus replies, "Let the dead bury their dead." And in parable he repeats this harsh requirement: "If any man come to me, and hate not his father, and mother, and wife, and children, and brethren, and his own life also, he cannot be my disciple."

The trouble with such absolutism is that it carries the seeds of its own corruption, and at the far end from Jesus' feeding of the multitudes, it echoes in Charles Taylor's enslaving of a generation of boys in Liberia by insinuating himself into the place of their elders. You can hear it in their 1997 campaign cry, the mockery of Christianity and democracy in a single slogan: "He killed my ma, he killed my pa; I'll vote for him."

———

The phrase "fictive family" sets me musing on the extreme idealization Tim displayed all his life, not just toward his father but toward his ancestors and all the permutations of family. There is little doubt that Tim transferred this intense loyalty to his soldier comrades in Hawaii, Europe, and Africa, and later to his de-mining teams. A guard among his trainees in Cameroon wrote "...we are proud of you because though still young you have proven that you are a good father.... You are for the truth..." An Ethiopian on his staff wrote after his death that Tim was "respectful and not just like a boss, it is just like father." His sister-in-law Ilke records that when she asked him why his men spoke so admiringly of him, he replied with a laconic "I'm tough but fair." Rob Jones proposed for his funeral program that he was "Once and forever part of that 'mysterious fraternity born out of the smoke and the danger of death.'"

———

That there is a very high quotient of bullshit in this notion of the fictive family does not diminish the loss when its promises are proven hollow. The solidarity of the brothers always rests to a certain degree on dehumanizing The Other. In our technological age, Marines use brutal video games to deform whatever image of honor or human feeling might make killing difficult.

Engorged with these speculations, I remind myself that Tim was drawn to the cheap and fragile toys of World War II before he could read, before we owned a television, before he suffered a concussion or endured his parents' divorce. Nor is there any doubt that the military offered him an adrenaline rush that could not be matched by the living room. Drawn to test himself to his limits, he was equally drawn to the rules that would place that daring in a noble system. Though it may seem that the yearnings toward risk and rules are at odds, and the ideas of hierarchy and community likewise, nevertheless that is what he sought and what the Army offered: extreme sport within an apostolic structure.

———

The Spartan code that provides the basis of the Western military (just as the Athenian court provides the basis of Western law) contains a stricture against unnecessary speech. The warrior isn't wordy. This part of the myth survives in our Westerns, our hard-boiled detectives and our national character. Loquacious and articulate in defense of his ideals, Tim subscribed to the Spartan model in matters personal and military. Because of this, it's impossible to know how much he knew of the failures, lies, and costs of the war he went to. He knew no WMDs were found, that Saddam had nothing to do with 9/11. He was aware that the RONCO Chief of Party for Eritrea—that is, his opposite number in the Ethiopian clearing operation—had come to de-mine in Iraq in May, been blown up and permanently disabled by a roadside bomb in July. He knew enough to speak of *corruption, lies, greed, and stupidity.* I don't know whether he realized that, in the words of Michael Gordon, author of *Cobra II*, "...our window of opportunity for the rebuilding of Iraq closed in summer 2003," by the time Tim arrived there. I don't know whether he saw the photos then circulating of Abu Ghraib or that RONCO had been accused of gun-running in Rwanda, that Pentagon audits would earmark $1 billion of Halliburton's invoices as "war profiteering," that hundreds of civilian contractor employees would die in the war—like the Iraqis, a form of collateral damage.

What I do know is that Tim, who had exasperated me through his teenage years by declaring, "My country right or wrong!" came at last heartbreakingly to say, "I'm ashamed to be an American."

———

In the event, the contractors stayed for the long haul, and are still there. Without their vast shadow army the Bush administration would have had to impose a draft, and the American people would not have stood for that. The Iraqi dead now number in the hundreds of thousands, and among American soldiers we have lost many more souls than on 9/11. Tens of thousands more carry their injuries through life. One in three returns from Iraq with a mental disorder and one in five with PTSD. In the meantime no one was tasked to keep records on either the huge sums entrusted to the multinationals or on the fate of the people they hired. By the time news of mercenary brutality and financial losses made its way through to the media, Americans had conflated the word "contractor" to mean both the multinationals and the people who worked for them, so there was no great incentive to keep track of the workers after they returned to their civilian lives. It will not be possible to count how many marriages end because of post-Iraq emotional problems, or how many children are emotionally maimed. As late as 2009 military officials told the Government Accountability Office that they "lacked a system" to track killed or wounded contractor personnel. The GAO had to go to the Labor Department to estimate through insurance policies even the number of people employed.

According to the Department of Defense, in 2010, 455 American soldiers died in combat, and a "minimum" of 407 by suicide. In 2012 there were more suicides than combat deaths. The Labor Department now estimates that one civilian contractor dies for every three combat soldiers. But there is no attempt to ascertain the number of suicides. Among the war dead of these American adventures, my son, literally, does not count.

———

Col. Ted Westhusing, U.S. Army Airborne, Ph.D. in philosophy from Emory University, professor of English at West Point, and one of the Army's leading scholars in military ethics, volunteered for deployment to Iraq in the fall of 2004. He thought the experience would help him to teach his cadets. In January 2005 he was assigned to the oversight of a private contractor training Iraqi security forces. In April his mood darkened; he worried about delays in the training. In May he received an anonymous letter detailing graft and human rights violations in the company. In emails to his family he grieved that the core West Point values had been replaced by profit motives.

In June 2005 Westhusing was found in his trailer at Dublin Base, the contractors' facility in Iraq, dead of a single shot from a 9 mm pistol. Beside him was a note in which he said, "I cannot support a mission that leads to corruption, human rights abuses and liars. I am sullied. I came to serve honorably and feel dishonored." It took the Army investigation three months to rule his death a suicide.

Tim had once told me, "…the warrior spirit…isn't directed at self and it isn't devoted to money. It needs an extreme integrity." I think Col. Westhusing was more intelligent, educated, and single-minded than my intelligent and dedicated son. But I think they were of the same mold and grieved over the same failures. Westhusing's father, Keith, says that "Ted was a loyalist, and, I believe, somewhat naïve in following his leadership in their reasons for going to war in Iraq….I had argued that they would not find WMDs….Ted told me: 'Don't worry. They'll find them.' He believed thoroughly in Honor, Duty, Country….The family has yet to understand this final act."

The military also had trouble understanding it. An Army psychologist assigned to review the case said, straight-faced, "Despite his intelligence, his ability to grasp the idea that profit is an important goal for people working in the private sector was surprisingly limited."

––––

Sgt. Michael Pedersen died a year before Tim, on April 2, 2003, when his helicopter crashed in central Iraq. In his last letter, he wrote his mother, Lila Lipscomb, that Bush had "lost the plot."

In July 2003, a month before Tim arrived in Iraq, Lance Corporal Jeff Lucey of the Marine Reserve returned from Iraq where, he told his parents, he had been ordered to shoot two unarmed prisoners of war. On the second order Lucey obeyed, watched the young men die, and then removed their dog tags and brought them home with him. He wore the tags until the night of June 22, 2004, when, two months after Tim's suicide, he hanged himself with the garden hose in the basement of the family home.

Specialist T.J. Sweet II, 23, shot himself with his M-16 rifle on Thanksgiving Day 2003. Tim had been in Baghdad nearly four months by then. On June 2, 2005, T.J.'s mother, Liz, helped a military honor guard lay a wreath for her son at Arlington National Cemetery. By that time Tim had been a year into eternity.

In March 2004, shortly after Tim left for home in Namibia, four American contractors were slain and burned in Fallujah: Stephen Scott Helvenston, Mike R. Teague, Jerko Gerald Zorko, Wesley K. Batalona. Two of their bodies were strung up over the Euphrates River. Parents of the four sued Blackwater Security for not providing them with the weapons they had been promised for their protection. But brother Jason Helvenston would not speak against the Iraqis. "We want to spread love for Scott right now and not hatred for others."

Casey Sheehan was killed in Sadr City on April 4, three weeks before Tim took his life. His mother, Cindy, camped out in Crawford, Texas.

On April 10, Tim with just two weeks to live, Justin Johnson, a First Cavalry machine gunner, was killed by roadside bomb. His 48-year-old father, Joe, joined the Georgia National Guard and went to Iraq to avenge his son's death. But he changed his mind. "I shouldn't have even come. If I go home and didn't kill a terrorist, it's not going to ruin my life. Maybe I'd just as soon not. I don't know what it's going to do to my head."

Pat Tillman was killed near the Pakistan border on April 22, the day before Tim killed himself, in what was originally presented as a heroic action, later friendly fire, later still a result of criminal negligence. His mother, Mary, said that she did not expect ever to get the true story of his death. "He watched his own men kill him...they lied about it..." At his funeral, his brother, Richard, said, "Pat Tillman is *not* with 'God'! He's fucking dead!"

Nick Berg, contractor, was beheaded in Iraq two weeks after Tim's death by a group of five kidnappers believed to be linked to al-Qaeda. Nick's father, Michael, blamed the murderers "no more nor less" than the U.S. administration. "Nicholas Berg died for the sins of George Bush and Donald Rumsfeld."

On June 13, 2004, National Guardsmen Lt. Andre Tyson and Spc. Patrick McCaffrey, training Iraqis to become military police, were killed at Balad north of Baghdad. Their deaths were reported as the result of insurgent ambush, but an investigation determined that they had been fired on by Iraqis attached to their patrol. Patrick McCaffrey's mother, Nadia, said that he had lost faith in the Iraq mission. "He was overwhelmed by the hatred there...he said we had no business in Iraq..."

Brigadier General Bernardo C. Negrete shot himself in front of his wife, Victoria, in their bedroom in San Antonio on September 16, 2005. His mother, Melinda Wingate, insisted it was an accident. "He loved life. There's no way he'd commit suicide." The medical examiner overruled her. "Look, we're not mind readers. All we know is, if you put a 9 mm pistol to your head and pull the trigger, we're going to call it suicide."

Spc. Joshua Omvig of the 339th MP company returned to his Iowa home from an eleven-month tour of Iraq and, on December 22, 2005, shot himself in front of his mother, Ellen, who declared him her hero and dedicated a website to her son and to "The War Against PTSD."

Spc. David Babineau was killed in the insurgent hotbed of Youssifah south of Baghdad and his companions, Pfc. Thomas Tucker and Pfc. Kristian Menchaca, kidnapped on June 16, 2006. Tucker and Menchaca were brutally tortured and beheaded, and responsibility was taken by al-Qaeda in Iraq. Tucker had left a message on the family answering machine: "I'm just gonna go on a little vacation, but I'll be back before you know it." Tucker's mother, Margaret, said, "There was no talking him out of it." His father, Wesley, added, "They are pawns of the politicians."

These are a few of whom I am aware.

And when I look up from my desk I still see among the pictures of those I love (CAUTION: THE WEARING OF HARD HATS IS REQUIRED ON THIS JOB), a grainy black and white image of an Iraqi father prostrate over the coffin of his son, with whom I have more in common than with the heroes of my own country, just as I have more in common with the mother of a Hamas suicide bomber who, dismayed at her grown son's political choices, is caught with no option but to let him go wrong-headed to his death.

13.

"It's nothing," I say to friends both before and after the procedure. "They put you out and feed a camera down your throat to see what's blocked."

And it's nothing. My esophagus has narrowed a tad, which causes the difficulty swallowing, and I suffer from a little acid reflux. The doctor stretches my elastic throat and prescribes the purple pill.

It's 2012. At morning "mucky talk" (so called because *mucky* was Anne's baby word for *blanket*), I describe for Peter the moment I went under the anesthetic. "I know, because the doctor asked me why I took Lyrica. Of course that's their trick. They want you to start talking, and then when you quit talking they know you're out." The point was that I knew too, in retrospect. I had said, "I have a neuralgia it took twelve years to diagnose..." I could precisely pinpoint my last word as "diagnose."

And I exist because I can remember the moment after which I no longer remembered.

This is what I struggle to convey over the cup of Colombian Breakfast Roast. But try as I might, because I cannot imagine not imagining, cannot think not thinking, cannot remember not remembering, I am. The brain, grappling with its own not-being, fails by definition.

"The trouble with dying," my brother writes,

"...is that everything dies. We lose not one loved one but all of them at once. We lose the kitchen table with the

161

*newspaper spread on it. We lose the half-empty jar in the
fridge and the memory of the jam we have eaten and the
anticipation of the jam that is left. We lose... the sight of
birds sliding on the wind. We lose the yellow line down
the center of the road... "*

To have suffered so near a death as that of a child puts you
in intimate connection both with the precious past and with
your very long future as *nothing*. Old songs and brutal news
make you bump up against the prospect of fatality; the face in
the mirror unflatteringly speaks of the sloughing of this mortal coil, but though religion labors to deny it, the passage *into,*
for yourself or your lost loved one, is fundamentally denied.

Under the leafing scuppernong vine I watch an ordinary
gray worm die. It's an inch or so long, segmented and noded
in miraculous camouflage as a twig. A quarter of the inch
is inert while the rest of it curls and writhes. I think maybe
it's caught under a splinter of the deck and so free it with
my ballpoint, but no, these are the throes, in full sun, being
performed just like this at this moment worldwide among
worms, crustaceans, amphibians, quadrupeds, and bipeds in
their millions. Next door, Mona's brother is being fed by the
hospice nurse. The worm arches, clenches, thrashes, and lies
still. Everything you and I know about death we have learned
by not experiencing it.

Unpleasant things come into my head and can't be sent
out again. A TV image of a prisoner eating a cockroach sits
on my tongue; a shadow in the doorway persistently conceals
a man in a balaclava. Don't think of... But this effort is the
opposite: a no-thing that cannot be brought to mind as long as
there is a mind to bring it to. I conjure a hole. Floating. Darkness. All of them are *something*, while I labor to birth oblivion.

On a photo beside this desk I have propped an insignia from Tim's uniform: AIRBORNE. I catch it in the corner of my eye and remember how he loved leaping out of planes. *One way or another you're going out. And you get to the door, it's your turn, and you go! And the silence you fall into is deeper than anything you've ever dreamed.*

Such silence!

Which, deeply, then, he heard.

Dare I say that this is also *interesting*? My mind chooses the painful exercise, just as my legs climb the elliptical machine, energetically going nowhere.

Imagine *nowhere*. Utopias notwithstanding, it can't be done.

————

What does it mean, "to heal"? What does it mean, "You don't get over it, you get used to it?"

A friend, in the first six months of forever after the death of her partner, is offended by the idea of healing. *It's a wound,* she says. *It doesn't heal; it can still open.* I refrain from pointing out that this is not the inevitable nature of a wound. She says that an acquaintance on the ditzy side of thoughtful sent her partner a box of healing stones and lucky feathers. For the atheist of New Age as of the Evangelical, magical trappings are offensive. The partner rejected them as "beach trash." And valiantly battled, though there is no ultimate outcome of this war except defeat.

Nor is there anything unusual about my grief—"this unique, banal thing," Julian Barnes calls it—or about my coming to live with it. We tend in America to look for change in epiphanic moments. We want the instant diet, the meteoric success, the Ravishing, an Aha! of healing. But *moving on* is not a sprint, and not really a triumph of the human spirit.

It is the doggedness of the world at your doorstep, doggedly knocking. One day you find you have read two consecutive paragraphs. One day you find you are angry not at the universe but at the local bank. One day you laugh, and quickly apologize to the beloved dead. One day a memory comes back shorn of grief, bearing only sweetness.

Rob Jones carried several shards of shrapnel in his legs and torso. He said he could go for long periods unaware of them. But bending a certain way he would feel the jab of alien metal. In extreme cold the edges sung. The loss of Tim is like that, still sharp although the scar has closed around it. Most of the time I move forward comfortably in an ordinary life. But sooner or later in the course of an ordinary day, I will happen upon a place, a person, a memento, and the shrapnel bites.

I offer my friend the image of embodied shrapnel, which she accepts, guardedly. It doesn't feel like the truth to her. At six months, the wound still opens.

———

Birgitt and Thyra immigrated and settled just outside of Atlanta, where we could drive up to spend the weekend, or they could drive down for holidays, beach, and pool. Thyra entered the same process of Americanization-by-school as her father had done thirty-five years before, and Birgitt began an immersion in the legal, political, and military convolutions of the Defense Base Act and the War Hazards Act, volunteer work that would keep her occupied for years.

Peter's Anne seemed ready to take hold of her life. She moved to Georgia and found a community of friends, including a boyfriend whose gentle patience drew her out of the anxiety that had long immured her. She took up photography and proved gifted at it. She made plans to become a nurse.

Peter bought her a used blue Acura that she babied with the care she had lavished on small animals as a child. She and Derek would join us for long evenings on the deck, to chat, eat, take photos of the owl and the raccoon who shared our backyard. Anne showed us the tattoo on her ankle: Tim's initials, a memorial in flesh.

In the summer of 2007 Peter and I went house-hunting in Wisconsin. It's hard in retrospect to credit how this came about—what we called "retiring backwards" to the north. We had amused ourselves for a decade choosing a retirement house wherever we went: La Jolla, St Augustine, Krakow, Eltville on the Rhine. We'd begun to say, half-joke, half-subtext, "I don't want to die in Tallahassee." My family was scant and far-flung but Peter's was large, concentrated in and around Milwaukee. We had been charmed the previous autumn by a 1927 fixer-upper in Lake Geneva—too seriously shabby, though, to take on the fixing.

That spring Alex and Trish were looking for a house in London, for prices that took our breath away. On a whim we checked the Internet to see what, for the price of a two-up/two-down south of the Thames, could be had in the Wisconsin woods.

I don't think there was any sense in which I needed to leave the house where Tim had grown up, but I do think I needed radically to change my life, rather than merely play it out. I was keener than Peter, but he was game. There was a sense in both of us of "now or never." We went up one weekend just to scout around, and came back with five bedrooms and five acres of Wisconsin forest, enough room to put up all the granddaughters and entertain Peter's Hungarian family. Anne and Derek said they would come up for Christmas in the snow. It was our adventure of the living room, and in truth we felt the apprehension of adventure. *Are you crazy?* people said. *You retire* to *Florida, not* from *it.* We signed the papers in August—at the exact moment that the market tanked.

We moved up the first week of October to fiery autumn, living like grad students with a bed, a folding table, and two folding chairs. We painted and scoured the antique stores, the furniture sales, scared but exhilarated because it felt like starting out.

Halloween evening I was sitting at the computer at the kitchen desk, procrastinating. I had judged a fiction contest and was putting off writing the email with my choice. At about eight, Peter's former wife, Jeanne, called in a mode he would later describe as "calmer than usual, unusually calm." Anne had been in an accident on the way to pick up Derek. She was hospitalized in Georgia but being flown back to Tallahassee Memorial. A "life flight," Peter told me, a term I'd heard only on TV. I did not immediately register its inverted meaning.

He went back to whatever game was on, pacing, however, unable to sit. Pacing, he said, "Jeanne always overstates."

I agreed. Nevertheless I went into my crisis-managerial mode. I wrote the email, "unusually calm," thinking, *I'd better get it done; I don't know what I may be doing later.*

I finished, and the wait became too long. I offered to call Tallahassee Memorial. Please, Peter said; he couldn't do it. I called, and was told Anne hadn't arrived yet, but they were expecting her. I found the phone numbers of two hospitals near Derek's home in Georgia, called the right one first, but was told that they could give out no information. Anne's mother was on her way and would call us when she got there. I said, "I thought they were flying her to Tallahassee Memorial." The nurse said, "No, that was the plan, but now they've changed their minds." And I was optimistic: no need after all for anything so drastic as a helicopter. Jeanne always overstates.

Peter said, "It's either good news or bad."

At once I knew Anne was dead. I said nothing.

But we waited. Waited. If Jeanne was driving up from Tallahassee, and the decision against the Life Flight had been between her call to us and mine to the hospital, how long would it take for her to get there, and how long after that to call? We talked little, and in retrospect the fact of waiting remains but the memory of it is gone. In any case, we waited. Then the phone tolled.

He said: "No-o-o-o-o!"

He said: "What do you mean we've *lost* her!? Do you mean she's dead!?"

He said: "I can't talk more right now. I'm going to hang up."

He hunched over the counter in a smart new swivel chair. I went awkwardly to him and awkwardly bent my body over his, like a hulking house, not comfort enough. He sobbed. I remembered how Alex had immediately cried at hearing of Tim's death, and again I envied that capacity.

———

We flew back to Tallahassee to lay her to rest (*What? In the ground!?*) and went through the formalities of death again. We added her name to the plaque on the park bench at Lake Ella that we had dedicated to Tim. The beloved blue Acura was totaled; we didn't want to see it. We rewrote our wills, again, and drove up to Moultrie, Georgia, for the accident report the insurance company required. Anne may have run a stop sign; she was hit in the driver's side by a van whose six occupants were drinking but were not much hurt. Her air bags did not deploy. The occupants of the van did not return to claim it.

We might have felt still more detached from Tallahassee, but what we felt in fact was: *too much disruption*. We took the house off the dismal market and rented it; we would be snow-birds until we got our bearings back. We traded in my natty Prelude for a snow-worthy four-wheel drive, and headed back to Lake Geneva.

We hadn't unpacked the car when our next-door neighbor called. She wanted to warn us: among the mail she'd taken in was a heavy box from Anne. I thanked her, prepared Peter, and brought it to him. The box held some twenty pounds of pecans that Anne had harvested at Derek's farm, with a note saying so, and love, and that she couldn't wait to see us in the snow at Christmas. From the postmark we saw that she had mailed it just before the post office closed, about two hours before she died.

———

Now it was my turn to be the rock. I had to learn that not everyone spills sadness in words, and that for Peter silence was soothing, distraction best. He took solace in routine, and food, and family. For a year we did almost nothing, drove through Wisconsin farmland, wandered the villages, tried this local restaurant and that, watched the bright fall and the enshrouding snow and the first unfurling leaf. I would look out into the beautiful winterscape, snow plopping from the branches, making divots in the smooth white coverlet, and ask: *Why have we lost two of our three children?* Because one lived with guns and the other, in Derek's words, "had a heavy foot and was easily distracted." Because we could take it. Because everybody has a short story or a long. Because death is certain and also arbitrary.

The statistics of survival for the marriage of a lost child are grim. We were "lucky," if that can be said, in that each of our children belonged to a former marriage, and so there was no impulse to blame each other for the loss of either. We were "lucky" in that the deaths occurred in tandem, so that each of us was able to be strong for the other. We were lucky—no quotes—in that we had each other.

And family flows into a void. We went in to Milwaukee for stuffed peppers with Peter's sister and for home-smoked fish with his niece; we fed them Peter's paprikash and my apple pie. We went after all to London to spend Christmas with Alex and his girls. We met and became close to Tim's sister Ana, acknowledging that we would never have met if it were not for his death. Birgitt and Thyra followed us up to snow country, and at this writing are living in the same Minnesota town as Tim's stepmother, Barbi, where we have visited them, dined with Barbi and her new partner, and watched Thyra punt a raft in the shallows of the lake where Tim and Alex did the same as children.

After two years, Peter took the pecans from the drawer where they had lain and buried them in the Lake Geneva garden.

Birgitt, having lost her own benefits case on appeal, continues to fight for contractors who are up against the same bureaucracy. She drafts legal arguments, puts victims in touch with lawyers, information sites, and each other; and collates information on the rise of PTSD. Thyra is still a popcorn machine, of increasingly American design. Neal the "undisciplined" works on a zipline in California while he takes a South African University degree online—but only after going through the world's stiffest discipline in Paris boot camp with the Foreign Legion. What this episode has to do with Tim we do not know, and do not suppose Neal knows, and have not asked.

Alex and Tricia are ensconced with the girls in their new South London house, where we continue to visit them every year, flying now from Chicago instead of the South. Alex manages a portion of the London Underground and in his spare time writes training manuals for international role-playing war games, full of his brother's vocabulary: *recruiting* and *missions* and *strategy* and *loadouts*. He tells me that his sense of loss increases rather than diminishes, that as the years pass he misses not only his brother but being a brother, living as what he never was or was meant to be, an "only child." Nevertheless, he writes, "I do feel that I've come to a peace with it. I do talk to him sometimes. Just the odd comment when I wish I could have shared something with him. There's little comfort in these vaguely melodramatic moments, but the repetition and rhythm of life draws you away from pain, and in its absence you heal. I think this is one of the reasons why humans are so drawn to music. It's a prehistoric attempt to imitate life and nature, and so to seek solace in that synergy."

Peter-the-lapsed-Catholic says, "God is omnipotent, omniscient, and omnivorous."

The public attitude toward contractors has not ameliorated, and if anything, has become more entrenched. Tim's name will not be carved on a granite wall or read out by Ted Koppel. The contractors are mostly, says *ProPublica*, "depicted as cowboys, wastrels, or worse." In the blogs, the *worse* runs from "war profiteers" to "no sympathy for these creeps" and "I would not cross the street to come to the aid of a merc." No one knows what it's like to be the bad man. The statistics on soldier suicide have forced that subject to the front pages, but in 2011 there were more suicides among contractors than among soldiers. "When the Pentagon farms out soldiers' work to contractors," says Rachel Maddow in *Drift,* "it not only puts more bodies in the field, it puts a different type of body in the field. The American public doesn't mourn the death of contractors the way we do the deaths of our soldiers. We rarely even hear about them."

A few years ago there was a vigil in Tallahassee. Little Lake Ella was to be surrounded by candles, one each for the dead soldiers of Iraq and Afghanistan. On the afternoon they were preparing, I went to the organizer, explained my mission, and asked if she could add a candle for my son. Of course. She wrote *Tim* in black felt tip on a paper bag, filled it with sand and wedged a little taper in the sand. At dusk I helped to light the candles. The lake covers perhaps six acres. The flames surrounded the whole of it, with inches between the bags. There were no speeches, no demonstrations, no taking of sides, just neighbors walking around the lake at dusk in shorts and sandals, with dogs, push chairs, children climbing the live oak for a better view. Later I must ask myself why, when I never wanted Tim to be part of the Army when he was alive, I was so comforted by his being included among the dead: the paper bag, the sand, the candle in the ring of light.

———

Grief is not the same as depression, can be in stunning ways its opposite. Depression leeches everything of joy, of purpose, of interest. I remember, depressed after my first marriage ended, thinking that the effort of putting my shoes on was more than I could bear. I shook through the aisles of grocery stores unable to buy milk, bread, meat. I lay on the floor unable to feel anything but the twisting of my stomach. I thought

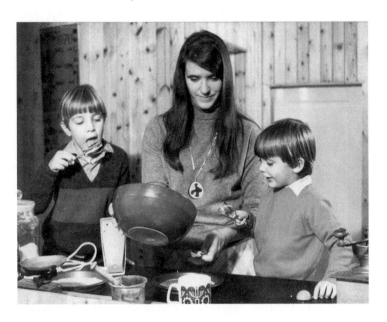

that everyone who seemed happy was merely duped. I was *unselved*. But for me grief does not operate that way. It can be intense. Ugly, awful, wracking. Intense. The things I've always enjoyed I still enjoy. The world still offers its extravagant haberdashery of beauty, boredom, love, and weather.

Walking one afternoon in the lush, familiar grounds of Paddington Rec in London—the roses, the gazebo, the playground, the cold cricket pitch—I saw that *loss* is another word for *longing*. At some point you realize that more of your life is behind you than ahead. You were told to "live in the moment," but you almost never did. On the contrary, the moments were tainted by wishing they would pass, or regretting the past, or anticipating something more wonderful. It's now, in retrospect, that their luminous significance is revealed.

Here, for instance, is a favorite photograph. In it I have just finished mixing a cake and am pouring it into two pans, having given the beaters to Tim and Toby to lick clean. A typical moment. Typically, Tim has gone right to it, while Toby is talking, talking, his free hand playing at a measuring spoon. The tea-towel calendar on the wall to the left behind us (Don't I still have the rag of that towel somewhere?) says 1970. We are all in sweaters, so it's either early in the year or late.

But wait. I'm wearing the only cashmere sweater I own, a heather-gray turtleneck, over a skirt I made from fine Italian wool with a muted pattern of diamonds, fabric I bought at John Lewis on Oxford Street, probably in the summer sales.

I don't wear that outfit to cook in.

So: 1970, a setup shot. Because I have saved (and carted across the Atlantic more than once) my daily calendars since 1959, I can find the day exactly. "23 November, 1970: 2:00 here—Ron Coburn, PR photos for ATV." A television play of mine was being sent to compete in the Monaco Festival, and the station was printing a brochure. (Don't I have that brochure in a file somewhere?) Tim is six-and-a-half in the picture, then, and Toby four.

It follows that the cake is a fake too, by way of Duncan Hines, but these boys have a theatre director for a father, and Tim has already appeared onstage as the son of the irrepressible Fenella Fielding in (cue irony) *A Doll's House*. We three know how to "act natural" for a publicity shot. All eyes are on the batter. Perhaps the cameraman has just said, "Smile!" and Toby and I are trying to comply without seeming posed. Tim does not interrupt his licking.

Center foreground is a mug whose blatant red-white-and-blue pattern leaps at me out of the photo grays. At extreme left and right of the foreground are an antique brass scale and a coffee grinder salvaged from Walter's grandmother in Ghent when I packed her up and moved her to the nursing home in 1964. She was placid, willing to go. I was considered to have the best temperament in the family to accomplish the move, and I probably had, which did not prevent me from a nervous fender-bender as I turned into her new home. By the time of this photo Walter and I regret all the things we let go to the parsimonious junk dealer (the stovetop waffle iron! the cabbage-shaped porcelain teapot!). All we have left of her now are the scale, the grinder, and a set of champagne glasses out of frame to the right, in the Welsh dresser built into the kitchen at its construction, on the countertop of which I stood barefoot, seven months pregnant with Toby, cleaning out cobwebs in the first days we spent in the house in September of '66. The distressed pine and the slate countertop are new. The floor is checkerboard yellow and orange, 1960s bright.

The bowl I'm holding is from Bennington Potteries, from our honeymoon visit in 1961. The peace-dove necklace was an anniversary present from Walter the next year, and has already had its ebony backing replaced, and within a little more than another year the wood will break again, and then I will somehow lose the dove (notice that the necklace is so designed that the bird is present by its absence) in the first few days of December 1971, the last few days before I take the boys and fly away with them.

Toby's sweater could be any Marks 'n' Sparks lambswool or hand-me-down, but Tim's I recognize as knitted for him by our sitter's mother, Auntie Cox, an outsize woman of outsize soul, who knits only in stripes because she uses up other people's leftovers or the hanks she salvages from discarded "jumpers." It is her theory that yarn, like flowers, goes together in any combination, and the boys have as yet developed no contrary opinion. Both boys sport the haircuts I gave them myself with a pride that I now see was somewhat misplaced. I cut my own hair, too, by drawing a part down the back, pulling the two resulting locks forward, and chopping each across with my sewing shears. I have trouble, now, remembering my hair was ever as long as that.

Out of sight to the left, between Tim's head and the calendar, is the kitchen window out of which I watch the boys climb sixty feet into the horse chestnut tree to pick their "conkers," my hands white-knuckled on the edge of the sink. Beyond that stands the little orchard, eight or ten trees we must have harvested last month and layered between newspapers in cardboard cartons that the local supermarket doles out grudgingly. Farther still, the road I take each morning, winding under the downs, dipping to the right into Ditchling village to drop Tim off at the ancient graveyard he must cross to get to his school, or to pick up Tricia who likes to be styled an "au pair" though she is an apple-cheeked local who grew up with Auntie Cox on a council estate; or rising left over the breathtaking Ditchling Beacon, rolling downs to the sea for one vista, crazy-quilt farmland for the other—on my way to Toby's pre-school and my office at the University.

Behind Toby's head is the door, as short as it looks, to the "wine cellar," a shelved nook into which we hunch, Walter to file or fetch his bottles, me to place or retrieve a pint of jam: raspberry, strawberry, black or red currant, goose- or lingon-berry, all of them from Mr. Ashley's abundant garden that grows behind you, past the table and the back door, over your right shoulder.

To Toby's right is the stove on which, one night when the university architect and his wife came to dinner and to advise us on the sinking floors, the broken windows, the defunct coal-fired furnace, I made a *béarnaise* sauce that Walter advised me on, tasted and tampered with, complained about, berated me for, until I took it past the table, to the W.C. beside the back door over your right shoulder, and poured it down the toilet. The architect's wife said, "Good for you."

Further right still is the door to the hall, wastefully large, and the staircase leading to the mezzanine from which Tim dropped his paratrooper G.I Joe, the steps he raced down in his stockinged feet, the one where he slipped and cracked his head, the fireplace where I built a fire and sat rocking him, rocking him as he spewed curse words and my breath came short with fear.

One photo. Left, right, up, down, to the past and farther past, to this person long lost track of, and back again: one photo. And I have hundreds—thousands?—of duplicates in boxes, a dozen albums kept up to the millennium, and an unedited plethora on the computer after that, each one of which can take me any direction, any distance, memory sparking memory that has no physical reality in the world, an unwritten fiction existing only in my mind, richer in detail and exactitude than any image of a future, rich with sorrow, precious.

And these memories, no snapshot required, also arise as ritual. If I go to sun on the deck in Tallahassee, I "place" Tim on the chaise. (If the chaise were gone I would resurrect it too.) He's in the pool teaching Anne to use the scuba gear, pulling scuppernongs from the pergola, flying baby Eleanor between his hands. Emotion flows from the fact of his absence and attaches gently to the repetition of the remembering. The repetition has the purpose of all ritual, which is: *remember this*.

There is no stilling of the inevitable *what-if*. If Anne had crossed that intersection thirty seconds earlier; if I had called Tim that Friday afternoon...but it is also possible, now, to feel that his life and hers are finished stories. Tim is no farther from me than he was in Africa, and in some ways nearer. I can imagine him as an adult in rooms he inhabited as a child, and in rooms now familiar to me that he never saw. I make him. I make him up.

———

Peter brings me my morning coffee and we settle in for "mucky talk"—Peter tells me about a friend he had, Bob Gansler, born in the same small village of Mucsi in Hungary, emigrated like Peter's family to Wisconsin, excelled in all sports, played minor-league baseball, then soccer for the Chicago Spurs and the Chicago Mustangs, coached the U.S. National Team in the World Cup in 1990, lost, played out his career coaching in Milwaukee, Kansas City, and Toronto, and was inducted into the soccer Hall of Fame early this century. "He was far and away better than the rest of us," Peter says. "A gifted athlete. I'll bet he made a difference in the lives of the kids he coached."

What strikes me is not anything to do with the man's career, but that dozens of times in situations casual or banal, in Tallahassee, Florida, but also in Vienna, Budapest, or Mexico, somebody who knew Bob Gansler half a century ago is talking to somebody who never knew him, saying: *He was great; I'll bet he made a difference.*

For those of us who don't believe in the coherence of the individual soul; for whom spirit, like matter, disperses silent into the universe, is it purpose and immortality enough to have displaced to good effect a certain space in the world for the period of our sentience?

For instance, this: there's a boy in—Boulder, Colorado, say—whose mother has come from Angola for a degree in computer science, who tells a friend about how this mother's family lived near the Namibian border when she was a girl, and they used to play along the power lines, where she didn't die because somebody had pushed the mines into berms and blew them up. And there's a hotel clerk in Addis Ababa, chatting to a minor diplomat from Venezuela, about how her grandfather's generation mostly perished in the Ethiopian–Eritrean wars, but he was born late enough that the border farmlands had been cleared. And there's a pregnant rug maker in Tikrit, one of six siblings in the textile trade, telling a merchant from Prague about how her great-grandfather used to play soccer in Taji West—a legendary athlete that boy was!—who won the heart of the smartest girl in town because he retained all four of his limbs, because in the American occupation that all the old people still remember, a particular kilometer of land was cleared of cluster bombs in 2003. And all over the world is a slender web in space and time, of people whose lives were changed, or who were born at all, because my son who loved weapons went, by the hazard of history, into the odd profession of getting rid of them.

And in that sense, there is no end to his story.

ACKNOWLEDGMENTS

If I were to list by name everyone who, in their kindness, insight and shared experience helped me toward the telling of this story, the acknowledgements would be as long as the book. It's a certain good in the discouraging state of the world, that friends rally, that family hunkers down, and that strangers open their arms and hearts. I would like to mention a few whose extraordinary generosity sustained me (and will certainly forget some, to whom I apologize): my son Alex Eysselinck and brother Stan Burroway, John and Blan McBride, Bob Butler, Elizabeth and Ned Stuckey-French, Pam Ball and Gary White, Elizabeth Dewberry, Joanna Goldsworthy, Joyce Ducas, Dolly Winch, Blair and Julia Kling. My husband Peter Ruppert was my rock.

When the obsessive outcries of my journal began to take shape as a book, I was encouraged and aided by a different set of necessary friends: my agents Emma Sweeney and Noah Ballard who encouraged me through many drafts; Adam Wahlberg who took on the task of publishing with great brio in chaotic times for publishers; artist Laurie Lipton who was asked to do a sketch of Tim and managed to include a dozen; author Jonathan Shay who has spent twenty years aiding veterans like my son Tim and offered to write the foreword; Ryan Scheife who designed the book from cover to cover, making old snapshots look fresh; and Kevin Finley, who took over the task of conveying the message not only to the usual literary suspects but also to veteran and suicide support groups around the country. In the process the manuscript was read and improved by the comments of excellent editors: Stan Burroway and Peter Ruppert again, Holly Carver, Madeleine Blais, Tom Jenks, Liz van Hoose.

My thanks to all of them, and especially to my readers, who by that act sustain a little of Tim's life.

RESOURCES

Wounded Warrior Project

The mission of the Wounded Warrior Project is to raise awareness and enlist the public's aid for the needs of injured service members; to help injured service members aid and assist each other; and to provide unique, direct programs and services to meet the needs of injured service members.

http://www.woundedwarriorproject.org/mission.aspx

National Suicide Prevention Lifeline

No matter what problems you are dealing with, the National Suicide Prevention Lifeline wants to help you find a reason to keep living. By calling 1-800-273-TALK (8255) you'll be connected to a skilled, trained counselor at a crisis center in your area, anytime 24/7.

http://www.suicidepreventionlifeline.org/

National Alliance on Mental Illness

NAMI is the National Alliance on Mental Illness, the nation's largest grassroots mental health organization dedicated to building better lives for the millions of Americans affected by mental illness. NAMI advocates for access to services, treatment, supports and research and is steadfast in its commitment to raise awareness and build a community for hope for all of those in need.

http://www.nami.org/

The Pathway Home

The Pathway Home is a healing community that bands together to embrace and assist the military personnel who have served our country in Iraq and Afghanistan. These service members have survived the stress of war, but find it difficult transitioning to civilian life because of the debilitating effects of Post Traumatic Stress, Traumatic Brain Injury, or other post-combat mental health challenges.

Intrepid Fallen Heroes Fund

Intrepid Fallen Heroes Fund is a non-profit organization that provides support to United States military personnel and their families. The fund began in 2000 and in 2003 was established as an independent not-for-profit organization.

http://www.fallenheroesfund.org/

American Contractors in Iraq

American Contractors in Iraq is made up of contractors, their families, and community members who aid in their efforts to keep contractors and their families up to date on issues that affect them now and in the future. Many injured contractors or family members of contractors find themselves fighting for the benefits that the Defense Base Act was intended to provide them.

http://www.americancontractorsiniraq.org/

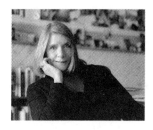

Janet Burroway is the author of eight novels and numerous plays, poems, essays, texts for dance, and children's books. Her novel *Raw Silk* was re-issued in 2014 by Open Road. Her *Writing Fiction: A Guide to Narrative Craft,* now in its ninth edition, is the most widely used creative writing text in America, and her multi-genre *Imaginative Writing* is out in a fourth edition. Her most recent novel is *Bridge of Sand* (Houghton Mifflin Harcourt 2009), and her play *Medea with Child* was produced in 2010 by Sideshow Theatre Company in Chicago. She has edited a 2014 collection of essays by older women writers, *A Story Larger Than My Own* (University of Chicago Press) and is at work on both a musical adaptation of Barry Unsworth's novel *Morality Play* and a play about her son. She is the Robert O. Lawton Distinguished Professor Emerita at the Florida State University and has been awarded the 2014 Lifetime Achievement Award in Writing by the Florida Humanities Council.